White Knight

Living with Alzheimer's Moment by Moment

Wanda M. Proost

ISBN-10: 1494370328
ISBN-13: 9781494370329

Dedication

Elijah Joseph Proost, I dedicate this book to you. Your grandfather was not able to watch you grow up. Grandpa will not be there for your Graduations, Birthdays, Christmases, or your Wedding Day. He will, however be with you in spirit. Grandpa had a big heart, Elijah and loved you and his children, unconditionally. His legacy is love. Love well, Elijah, be his light in this world. When life throws you a curve, when you can't feel your feet. "Remember to look up and live your life moment by moment. Grandpa will be there with you."

My second dedication is to all caregivers. May God bless all of you. I know how you struggle, cry alone at night, and worry if you are doing enough for the one you love. I know you are tired. Rest assured you are not alone. The hole in your heart will be filled with love and God's grace. It is a unique gift to be a caregiver and you are a blessing to your loved ones. Fill your lives with love and laughter and live every day, with grace and dignity. Slowly you will climb back up those stairs moment by moment and you will be healed.

This last dedication is to Cheryl Proost and closest to my heart. Cheryl, you have been a blessing to me. We have traveled long and far together. Our lives have brought us great joy and deep sadness. You were there for me as I traveled down that long staircase with Joe and you were there helping me climb back up that same steep staircase. You have endured hours listening to me, advising me and cheering me on as I wrote this book. I love you. I pray that you and I will have many more adventures and that we can continue to live our lives in light and love.

Forward

*I*t came as a complete surprise when my sister-in-law and close friend told me she was writing a book and more of a surprise that she was writing about Joe. Joe was my husband's fraternal twin brother. I introduced Wanda to Joe at the boys fiftieth birthday party and they were married a couple of years later.

Theirs was a love story touched by tragedy. As you will read, after six years of marriage, Joe was diagnosed with early Onset Alzheimer's. You will find yourself engulfed in the emotional and traumatic events of their lives, page by page.

Not only has Wanda written a beautiful love story but a guide for every caregiver taking care of a loved one. Her stay-in-the-moment attitude works equally well for caregivers in hospitals or at home with their patients.

Many life-changing events happen in the blink of an eye; car accidents, heart attacks, natural disasters, personal attacks and the results are immediate. With Alzheimer's, the effects and the ramifications happen over time. You lose your loved ones slowly one day at a time, moment by moment. There is no road map for caregiving with this disease; however, there are basic similarities between patients.

Wanda's insight gives hope to those who bear the heavy responsibility of watching their loved ones slowly lose themselves. Joe had to rely on Wanda for everything. She made all decisions and the task was enormous. Because, they were still so young, she had to work while taking care of Joe. She was tireless in her efforts to insure Joe and everyone that interacted with him, was comfortable and at ease. Wanda made caregiving look easy however, in reality it was not.

As Joe's disease began to progress, he would not let her out of his sight. She was his anchor. I prayed for a miracle and instead found the miracle in the process. We all began to live in the moment with Wanda and Joe; this process enriched all of our lives.

Wanda shows the reader how to live well, how to see the positive and live with the faith that miracles happen daily in the small acts of love and kindness, life is in the ordinary moments.

My name is Cheryl Proost and I am proud to recommend this book to anyone faced with the enormous task of caregiving. I lived this disease with Wanda and I can tell you from personal experience that living moment by moment will change your life and the lives of your loved-ones immeasurably.

With Heartfelt Love,

Cheryl

Introduction

*A*lzheimer's disease is a progressive, degenerative disorder. It is estimated that 5.1 million Americans may have Alzheimer's, and about half a million Americans younger than sixty-five have some form of dementia including Alzheimer's.

It is estimated that one to four family members act as caregivers for each individual with Alzheimer's. These facts have come from the Alzheimer's Foundation of America.

My husband was diagnosed with Early On-set Alzheimer's. Four years later he died in a convalescent hospital. This is our story.

Before you begin reading, I want to explain a few things about this book. First, the stairs on the cover are a metaphor; I see them as the stairs of life. Babies climb the stairs of life as they begin to learn and understand their place in this world. When they reach the top, they have grown into adulthood. Alzheimer's patients descend those stairs as they lose understanding and their place in this world. When they reach the bottom, they have passed out of our lives.

The title of this book; *Living with Alzheimer's, Moment by Moment,* is the way I coped with my husband's debilitating disease. I had no choice but to live with it. I found that by staying with Joe in his moments made my moments not only tolerable but also enjoyable. I found that by leveling my emotions with his and feeling each moment, I bypassed a lot of pain and suffering on my part. I also began to notice that his response to me became a smooth flow of love and he seemed to relax into his situation with ease and fluidity, as did I.

My experience with Joe was surreal and poignant. I mourned for the husband he once was, more importantly, I mourned the way he made me feel about myself. I was mourning the loss of me as a woman and his wife. There were days when I completely forgot he was sick, then, as I remembered, I would cry for the loss of him. I write this book to give other caregivers hope.

I will show you how I made the most of the many blessings I received. I will explain to you how I stayed in the moment with him. I want you to see this disease in a new and wondrous way, as I began to see Joe in a new and wondrous way. Life is a journey and who is to say how that journey unfolds; everyone's story will be unique. Your outlook on a situation determines the experience of that situation.

I lost myself and immersed myself in this disease. My every waking thought was for Joe and his well-being. However, after he died, I came back stronger than ever. My life had a new purpose. As with all lessons in life, this journey was not always easy.

I look at myself in the mirror now, realizing that Alzheimer's has taken so much from me, but gave me so much more. I am stronger and I continue to stay in the moment. I use the gift Joe gave me to savor life in its ever changing tides. I feel blessed and honored to have known, loved, and cared for him every single day.

The beginning of each chapter starts with either a quote from Joe or a poem from me. We wrote to each other every day while Joe was in Iowa. These letters and poems have provided me with rich fodder for this book.

I began our story in the middle, when Joe first went to the doctor. I used dream sequencing to catch the reader up on our lives from the beginning, indicated by dates, so as not to confuse you.

My wish for you, the reader is that if even a small part of our story can have a positive impact on your journey I will have been successful and Joe's legacy will live on. Stay in the moment and feel each moment with your patients. Try to see the world through their eyes. Notice the many blessings they bring to your daily life, love them for who they are at any given moment and God will help with the rest.

As with all love stories, they start with Once upon a time...

In love, Wanda

one

Joe

You opened up my eyes.
You helped me see your glory.
You helped me see my glory.
You helped me smell the sea.
You helped me smell the flower.
You let me touch your heart.
You opened up my eyes.
You let me feel your love.
You let me feel your pain.
You let me taste your tears.
You helped me taste my tears.
You let me touch your heart.

Wanda

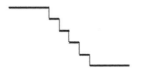

O nce upon a time, in a land not far away but long forgotten, there lived a White Knight with his lovely young bride. They lived together in the dark green hills near the calm blue ocean, loving each other, they tasted every moment and it was sweet. They frolicked in the lush landscape and swam naked in the calm, cool surf. They made love in the soft moonlight.

One day the Knight was stricken with a strange disease that no doctor of the land could cure. Each one came, shook their heads, then left saying there was nothing they could do. Near death, the White Knight lay on his bed with his devoted wife by his side.

The Knight took her hand in his and stroking the inside of her right wrist with his thumb said, "Never fear my dear wife; I will see you again soon, real soon."

"But, how will I know you?" the distraught wife cried.

As the Knight took his last breath and continued to stroke her wrist he whispered, "Don't worry, you'll know me."

With that, the young wife covered her beloved Knight with her cloak as she lay down beside him. They looked lovingly into each other's eyes as he let out a sigh of love and peace and was gone.

The lonely young wife, filled with the love of her White Knight spent the rest of her life spreading peace and hope to everyone in the land.

FEBRUARY 2005

Joe and I stood on the sidewalk next to our car; we held each other so tight that we could feel our hearts beating. We cried in long tormented sobs, tears streaming down our faces, we did not attempt to wipe them away. Our lives changed today irrevocably, never to be the same.

Joe finally stepped back from me, took my face in his big strong hands and said, "Wanda I'm so sorry to be such a bother. I'm very worried that you'll spend your life taking care of me. I'm not concerned about me; this isn't fair to you."

I whispered back, "I will always take care of you, Joe. We'll do this together with grace and dignity."

He kissed me then long and hard, his familiar lips on mine drinking in my essence. We were oblivious to the traffic on Freedom Boulevard. Cars streaming past us held drivers going about their normal day. The sun was shining, white puffy clouds hung like sentinels in the pure blue sky. I could only see Joe.

Our lives now held in suspended animation, while the rest of the world continued to move on without us. Our journey would take us down the stairs of life. I would become Joe's caregiver; he would become my greatest teacher, I his student.

I was desperate to get to Jim and Cheryl's house, Joe's brother and sister-in-law. I needed to give them the results of our doctor's visit; we needed them more now than ever. As I drove, I flashed back to my first meeting with Joe.

MARCH 1997

Cheryl was planning a 50th birthday party for Jim and as a surprise she sent Joe, Jim's twin brother, a plane ticket so they could spend their special day together. When I heard that Joe was coming I was a little curious, but nervous as I knew Cheryl was expecting us to make a connection. Joe had been divorced from his wife of twenty years for four years and was living alone in Minnesota. I will always be grateful to her for that first introduction; she changed our lives forever.

I woke up with nervous anticipation in the pit of my stomach. As I got dressed for the party, I tried to guess what Joe would look like, would he have Jim's thick white curly hair and piercing blue eyes. Would he be as outgoing as Jim? I actually had to laugh; ok maybe I was a little excited.

I had not considered meeting another man; I had been married for twenty-five years and now divorced for two. What should I say, how should I act? I spent extra time on my make-up and hair, I chose my clothes carefully; I wanted to look great, conservative, but a little sexy. I wore a black printed blazer, black tights, and black boots.

I arrived a little late and the party was in full swing. Cheryl had invited all of their closest friends. I barely got through the front door as Cheryl scooped me up and took me over to Joe.

She was so excited that she could barely get out the introductions. "Wanda, this is Jim's twin brother Joe; Joe, this is Wanda, Amy and Abby's mother."

"Hi Joe, it's great to meet you." I said, stomach churning.

Joe reached for my right hand and began to stroke the inside of my wrist as he said, "Wanda, it's wonderful to meet you, Jim and Cheryl have told me so much about you."

The rest of the day was spent in a sort of dance, mingling with all of the guests, but never out of sight from one another. As I snuck glances at him, I wondered what it would be like to know him. There was an instant connection between us; we could both feel it. I knew I was having a "once in a lifetime experience."

As Jim and Joe began cutting their birthday cake, I had eyes only for Joe. He stood there with thick black hair, cut short, square jaw, ruddy complexion, light blue eyes, sturdy body and all I could think was; he is going to be my husband! I felt an immediate tug at my heart. This was an "outside the box" experience for me, unexpected, but not unwelcome.

Joe came up to me as the party ended, took me in his arms and gave me a full body hug whispering in my ear, "I will see you again soon real soon!"

My breath caught in my throat, my legs weak; I did not have the strength to answer him. I looked in his soft baby blue eyes and smiled. The party now is a blur; all I see when I look back on that day is Joe's eyes, he magnetized me with those eyes.

FEBRUARY 2005

We pulled up to Jim and Cheryl's house just as they arrived. I snapped back to the present and the sad task of telling them that Joe was sick, with either Mad Cow Disease or Alzheimer's. I was scared and panicky; I could feel our lives crumbling.

"Hi Joe, how are you?" Jim said in a relaxed but serious tone.

Joe answered, "Good Jim, how are you?"

Jim kept his head down and headed for the house, we followed slowly behind him, once inside Jim asked. "So, what's up?

I shakily recounted the doctor's dire prediction, tried to explain Joe's symptoms, and answered their many questions. Joe was having difficulty remembering his social security number, which he used to punch the time clock at work. He could no longer tell time. Joe had trouble identifying his co-workers and got lost at work. He did not know his address or phone number or what day it was or what time it was. Joe could not use his power equipment. He did not know his birthday.

Jim and Cheryl sat there in abject silence. Finally, Jim put his head in his hands and wept. Cheryl and I let tears of disbelief slide silently down our faces. Joe tightened his grip on my hand; his face was devoid of emotion.

Joe finally spoke up and said, "I'm so sorry about all of this, I don't know what to do, please don't cry, I'll be alright; it is what it is."

Jim quickly regained his composure and said, "Come on Joe let's go outside and take a walk."

"Ok, Jim do we have a project?"

"I'm sure we can find one, we can always cut the lawn." Off they went; no two brothers were closer they loved each other and needed each other so much.

Cheryl, my darling sister-in-law and close friend and I headed to the kitchen. Her lips quivered as she asked me, "What are you going to do?"

"Joe's doctor has scheduled an appointment with a neurologist for next week; then he will be scheduled for a brain scan and blood work."

My mind had slowed to a crawl, I felt like I was buzzing, "I don't know Cheryl; I guess we will see what the tests reveal and then move forward one day at a time, our lives were so perfect, this can't be happening!"

I began to cry. Cheryl moved from behind the counter, took me in her arms, and let me cry on her shoulder.

"Please don't cry Wanda, I can't stand it, you're making me cry. You're the strong one don't fall apart on me. Jim and I will do whatever we can to help you with Joe."

"I know you will." I stepped away wiping my eyes, I needed to pull myself together. I did not want Joe to see me like this.

"Cheryl, I have to go back to Joe's office to get disability paperwork and take it to his doctor, will you come with me? I don't want to be alone."

"Yes, let me get my purse, the boys are busy in the backyard they'll be fine, while we are out we'll get dinner, I don't feel like cooking."

"Good idea, I don't feel like eating, but I know nothing will stop Jim and Joe from dinner, we should get a great desert, maybe chocolate cake and ice cream."

Cheryl and I drove to Joe's office in silence; lost in our own thoughts. Life for me was a roller coaster filled with highs and lows; it looked like the Richter scale. I almost was not surprised at this turn of events.

My marriage had been hard; the decision to divorce even harder. Giving birth to identical twin daughters had been so much fun, albeit challenging; Amy and Abby were the frosting of my life. My children always provided me with hours of entertainment!

Joe burst on the scene like a White Knight in Shining Armor. Everything about us was perfect; we fit together in every way. Never a day has gone by that I did not thank God for all my many blessings. Now this, I knew Joe did not have Mad Cow Disease; he would have had to eat the brains of an infected cow. Early Onset Alzheimer's; I did not know much about this insidious disease. Tomorrow I would buy a book to see what we were up against; being an avid reader, I would read it cover to cover.

After a delicious dinner of steak, baked potatoes and chocolate cake, Joe and I headed home. We were both exhausted, but too tired to sleep. Joe took me in his arms and made passionate, slow sweet love to me. Later, as we lay in each other's arms I cried, filled with such love of him, there were no words.

Joe's deep breathing signaled sleep; I spent most of the night awake, my mind wandered back to our first Christmas together.

two

Loves Blooming

Standing in my fertile mind, I see the rooms of
my past, very familiar, very sad.
I look at each piece of myself and I feel the old feelings, always
tinged with melancholy, tears always on the fringe.
I gently say good-bye to my old feelings putting
everything to rest, the guilt, the sadness, the pain.
I can do that now because of you, because of the sheer wonder of you.
You have taught me to see the present, to let go of the past, not bury it.
I now see the future, moment by moment and I'm at peace.
I'm happy for the first time in my life, because
of your sweet and gentle spirit.

Wanda

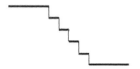

DECEMBER 1997

The phone rang at Amy and Andon's house December 22 at 6pm. I was watching my first little granddaughter; her mom and dad had gone out to dinner. Bailey was running around the house, in a white t-shirt and a very dirty diaper.

I was getting her ready for bed as the phone rang; it was Jim. "Hey! My brother Joe is back in town. We picked up a pizza and a movie. We will be over in ten minutes!"

It had been a crazy month, getting ready for Christmas, this call made my heart stop. I had not heard from Joe since I met him in March at the birthday party! I looked at myself in the mirror, Oh God! I think I looked worse than Bailey! Whom do I clean up first? We only had ten minutes Bailey won! I hoped that I would smell better if Bailey did. I changed her dirty diaper and put her in warm cozy pink pajamas. I threw on some of Amy's perfume, ran a brush through my short, curly black hair, a little mouthwash and the doorbell rang.

My heart skipped a beat as I opened the door to the most handsome man in the world. Joe stood there with a big grin on his face and a pizza. He put the pizza down and took me in his arms. I melted into another full body hug, I felt like I was home!

"Hi Wanda, I'm back and so happy to be here with you!" he whispered

"Oh, Joe!" I moaned.

He walked through the door and into my life. We sat on the couch eating pizza and watching a movie. Bailey would not leave my lap; she kept looking over at her great Uncle Joe. I know she was wondering who he was and why he was sitting so close to her Granny! Cheryl and Jim kept up a lively chatter to compensate for Joe's and my stinted silence. As the movie, progressed Joe kept slipping closer pressing his thighs to mine. I will never forget the way my body reacted to him.

FEBRUARY 2005

Joe was sleeping peacefully; I put my head on his chest and finally fell into a dreamless sleep, eager to put the day's trials behind me. I awoke with a start; it was still dark outside. Joe standing at the foot of our bed stark naked had banged on the bed with his knee to wake me.

I groggily sat up as he said. "Get up its almost first light we don't want to miss the sunrise, come on coffee is ready!"

He almost jumped into his jeans and an old blue sweatshirt as I stumbled to the bathroom, "Oh Joey, really?"

"Yeah, come on coffee on the patio!"

I had to smile as I looked at my puffy eyes from a night of crying and tousled black hair, it was amazing that he could love me, sometimes I really believed love was blind.

We sat on our patio and watched the sunrise sipping steaming hot coffee. For a moment, I almost forgot about yesterday and the doctor's dire diagnosis. Joe chatted happily about politics, the yard and the day that stretched before us. I had to get ready for work.

"Today Joe you don't have to go to work."

"Why not?"

"Because you are on vacation, you get to stay home with Riley."

Riley was our Scottish terrier; Joe had bought him for me soon after we moved in together.

"I will leave lunch in the refrigerator and I'll be home about six, I'll cook dinner. Oh, by the way don't drive today, ok?"

"Why not?"

"Because until the doctor tells us what is wrong with you, no driving!'

Joe said in very good humor, "Alright, I will be busy here all day, but I'll take Riley for a walk."

"Ok, just stay in our subdivision."

With a deep sigh Joe said, "Ok! Boy, what is wrong with you?"

"Nothing!" I said under my breath as I walked back to the bathroom to take a shower.

I let the hot water run over my still sleepy body, trying to get my bearings. Should I tell my boss about Joe, maybe he might have some good advice. I could hear Joe rattling around the kitchen; I wondered what he was making for breakfast, probably cereal.

Cold cereal, he was so sweet! I gulped down breakfast, raced for the door and a quick kiss for Joe. I snatched the truck keys, no driving for him today!

Traffic was slow and again my mind began to wander, back to that first Christmas.

DECEMBER 1997

Christmas Eve dawned sunny and bright. I stayed in bed a long time before rising, my head dizzy with anticipation. Amy and Andon; my daughter and Cheryl and Jim's only son were hosting tonight's festivities. I was very nervous because my whole family was going to be there including my ex-husband, Lloyd. Lloyd and I had remained fast friends since our divorce. It seemed right somehow, we had so many people we loved in common. I relied on him for his advice on many issues. I never wanted to hurt him in any way so today would be a challenge. I had not shown interest in any man since him and I was concerned how my budding relationship with Joe would affect our easy relationship.

I could not imagine how this night would play out. I spent the day before preparing dinner; I usually cooked. Finally, it was time to get ready for the "big" show; my movements were wooden. I fumbled with my make-up, my jewelry and doing my hair. Funny, the world seemed to slow to a crawl, as my heart beat wildly!

I was a little late to show up, food in hand, everyone met me at my car to carry in the many pans of chicken enchiladas, rice and beans. By the time I made it to the front door, I was sweating.

"Hey, where have you been? You're late; we need to get the enchiladas in the oven now!" Everyone chimed in at once.

I flashed a sheepish grin, "I'm so sorry it took forever to get this food in the car!" I lied.

The house was warm and cozy with a big tree gaily decorated with bells, bows and lots of tinsel. The house was crowded with all of my family. It was a night filled with laughter and teasing. Joe made a big impression on everyone, he was engaging and very charming; no one guessed the connection between us except

Lloyd. It became a tug of war as to who could get closer to me, Lloyd or Joe.

After a very lively and entertaining dinner, we began the three-hour process of opening presents. My dad, who was always the star of the show at Christmas, donned his "Santa Hat." He always played Santa Claus and expected us to open presents one at a time. Dad was so cute and very funny, before long the whole house was in stitches. After presents, we ate homemade apple pie and ice cream for dessert.

Joe came up behind me, gently pressing his body up against me and whispered in my ear, "Do you want to go to a party with me and Jim and Cheryl tonight?"

"Yes!" I said with no hesitation. I had always spearheaded the cleanup and wondered how my girls would take my desertion.

As we said our good-bye's I could hear my dumbfounded girls saying, "Where is mom going, who is going to clean up this mess?"

I laughed to myself all the way to the car. Tonight, I felt like a grown up and a little bit sexy!

I drove with Joe sitting next to me in the front seat. Jim and Cheryl sat in the back. Jim and Joe kept us entertained with stories of their high school years. I kept thinking to myself, what are you doing, Wanda? I could not believe Joe was here and now I was out with him. My heart beat fast as I contemplated my future, which would include Joe.

MARCH 2005

I pulled into my office parking lot after what seemed like a very short drive, daydreaming and driving, not a good combination. As I walked into the office, I still had not decided whether to tell my boss about Joe.

He was a wonderful man, kind and compassionate. We always met before we saw our clients for the day. I was the office manager, and intimately involved with all aspects of his company. Today, I had decided not to tell him about Joe. I was not ready for his reaction; I had only worked for him about six months and was scared he would let me go.

I had just sat down as he burst through the door to my office.

"Good morning, we have a busy day, how are you, ready to go?"

"Yes, I'm ready; we have four clients before lunch." I said in a wooden tone.

"Are you sure you are alright, you seem upset?" he queried.

I said nothing; put my head down and much to my embarrassment burst into tears. He stopped for a moment, then got up out of his chair, came around to my side of the desk and pulled me into his arms. I stood there and sobbed on his navy blue silk blazer.

After a few minutes, he let me go, looked me in the eyes, and again said, "What is wrong?"

"Oh my God! Joe is sick; the doctor thinks it is either Mad Cow Disease or Early Onset Alzheimer's. We went to the doctor yesterday and will see a neurologist next week. I was afraid to tell you, as I haven't been here very long. I don't want you to let me go, I'll still be able to do my job!" I choked.

"Whoa, whoa! Slow down you're not going to lose your job."

He sat there in my office in stunned silence as I told him about Joe. I could barely speak struggling to hold back my tears.

When I finished, he quickly spoke and said, "I'm so sorry. Wanda, you are not in danger of losing your job. You're doing great and I need you. I'll do anything I can to help you. As you get information you can talk to me, I have broad shoulders! If you need time off for doctors' appointments just let me know. I'm so sorry Wanda; this is going to be rough!"

"Thank you," I said wiping my eyes.

"Take a few moments, our first client can wait a few minutes." My boss said as he headed back to his office with a slow step and a heavy heart.

"Ok, I'll be right there."

three

Seeing

When someone asks a question, does she really want an answer?
When someone poses a problem, does she really want a solution?
When someone has an idea, does she really put it to use?
When someone looks at the world, does she really see what's there?
When someone looks within, is she really searching for the truth?

Wanda

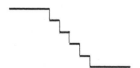

I told my mother, sisters, brothers, and children about Joe and each time I cried. I could not see how anyone could help me. They consoled me, asked what they could do and I always said, "Nothing, I'll be all right". However, I was not all right, I was in pain.

I have always looked on the bright side; my typical Pollyanna approach to life had always been I could do anything. However, this time, inside I was pleading, "Can't you hear me screaming?" I had experienced major problems in my life and I did not complain, quite the opposite I always stood up and made the best of every situation. I was absolutely committed to that same attitude now.

This time, when I really needed help I crawled into myself with Joe. My love for him was so strong that I was insistent on giving him as much quality and normalcy in his last years as possible. Joe had given me the most wonderful gift of love; now it was my turn to return that love in spades. I believe that as he danced into Heaven he took the only thing I had to give him, love.

After two brain scans, a spinal tap, and many blood tests all sent to the Mayo clinic, Joe's neurologist, called us and wanted us to sit before a panel of 20 doctors. He was hesitant to render a diagnosis of Alzheimer's because Joe was so young; he wanted other opinions. I agreed.

We arrived the next day to an audience of Doctors, men and women, most had coffee all looked relaxed and were talking amongst themselves. They acted as if it was just another day at the office; to me it was a nightmare. Our doctor, Joe and I sat in chairs lined up on a stage. The panel sat in front and below us. Joe's doctor had put the results of the CAT scans on a viewing screen to our left. The conversation began with a dissertation from Joe's doctor outlining the tests done and the results.

Then the doctors began to talk to Joe. He was happy, engaging and laughing. He acted as if he was at a party.

As they began to question me, they asked, "What was Joe like before he began experiencing memory problems?

I answered in a clear, strong voice, "Joe was intelligent, interested in politics, history and was loving, kind and very sensual. In college, He was a springboard diver and almost made it to the Olympics. Joe had a successful career in sales. In the last few years before he got sick, his interest turned to construction; he was a very skilled woodworker and could fix almost anything. Joe studied and received his class B contractor's license with ease."

"What can he do now?" A doctor in the front row asked.

"Now, nothing on his own; he waits for direction from me. Joe follows me everywhere. Getting dressed on his own; is hard for him. He eats on his own, but needs supervision, as he is beginning to have problems deciding which utensils are appropriate. He still enjoys music and dancing. He loves gardening, however, cannot use pruning shears." My voice began to crack as I was forced to admit how far Joe had fallen into his illness.

Joe's doctor rescued me from the questions of these curious doctors; he realized I was about to cry. "Let's wrap up these questions. What do you think about Mr. Proost's diagnosis?"

Finally, after much discussion amongst the panel, one doctor in front stood up and said, "We have been over the results of all the tests, it is clear by the MRI that Mr. Proost's brain has shrunk to that of an eighty year old man. We have questioned the patient and his wife, we have no choice but to render a diagnosis of Early On-set Alzheimer's; there is nothing we can do."

All of the doctors agreed and began leaving the room; some of them came up to me shook my hand and expressed how sorry they were. Five minutes later, we were alone on the stage, I could not move.

Joe's doctor said, "Come back to my office, I want to talk to you." We slowly left the stage and followed him back to his office.

One of the nurses sat with Joe engaging him with books, as I walked with leaden legs back to his doctor's office. "Sit down, Wanda I am sure you have many questions and I have some things to tell you."

My first question was, "How long does Joe have to live?"

He answered in a very direct manner, "Early Onset Alzheimer's usually goes quick, probably about two years."

I gripped the arms of the chair and in a barely audible voice, said, "Two years? That is too soon; I'm not done loving him yet! Is there anything we can do? Are there any drugs that will help?"

Joe's Doctor said in a resigned voice, "There are some drugs that will slow the process, but nothing that will cure him. Before we discuss what kind of drugs to give Joe, I want you to know something. If you decide to give him the medications, they will only prolong the process. Drugs will not cure him, they may improve the quality of his life in the short term, but they will only prolong his disease. Do you understand me, are you willing to do this, your situation will last longer Wanda, do you understand?"

I sat there in stunned silence, unable to speak.

"I want to tell you what you can expect from Alzheimer's; Joe will continue to lose the present, and soon he will forget the past. He will be unable to recognize family and friends. Joe will need constant care and he'll continue to have trouble dressing and feeding himself. Eventually Joe will forget who you are, although that will come last, as he is so attached to you and you are his primary caregiver."

"Alzheimer's patients tend to be wanderers; they often have sleep problems and will be up at night when you are trying to sleep. Sometimes, patients become scared and can lash out at their loved ones. Eventually they forget how to walk, talk and eat. They become bed-ridden and usually die of pneumonia."

I felt the blood leave my face, my mouth went dry and I could barely breathe. Joe's Doctor got up from his chair and came to my side; he put his hand on my shoulder to comfort me.

This was unbelievable; I could not wrap my brain around his words. I felt like I was drowning, silent tears began to slide down my face.

"What can I do now?"

"Go home and love him, you still have some time, this will happen slowly, please think about the drugs and let me know.

"I don't have to think about the drugs, yes please start him on them today!"

"Ok, but, please remember what I said, this drug will not stop this disease, only prolong it." He said in a very serious tone.

"If our situations were reversed, Joe would do this for me, I have to try!"

"I wish I had better news. I know how much you love him and it is obvious how much he loves you. Joe is lucky to have you."

I bowed my head, looking at my feet. "Thank you for everything." I said.

"You call me if you have any questions day or night."

"I will."

With that, I rose from my chair on wobbly legs and headed for the lobby and my wonderful happy child/husband.

Joe's face lit up when he saw me, he rushed up to me and grabbed my hand and I kissed him lightly on the lips.

"Can we have a treat?" he asked.

Treat to Joe was mocha. I said, "Yes, I want mocha too!"

Joe slept in the car on the drive home. My mind was reeling; I could not believe that in a couple of years, this man who slept so peacefully beside me would be gone. This man who charged into my life like a White Knight in Shining Armor capturing my heart and soul would no longer share my life. How unfair this was, how terrifyingly sad, I was missing him already. How would I live without him, how could I face a day without experiencing first light with him? How could I look up at the moon at night knowing that he was not seeing it with me?

I had many calls that afternoon from family and friends. As I recounted the morning's events, I would break into sobs, and they would say they were sorry; they would be there for me and then hang up. I was alone with Joe, alone with him in our moment of pain.

We went to bed early, I was exhausted and I had to go to work the next morning. I lay on his chest feeling him breathe; overcome by the blessing of his presence. Someday in the not too distant future my bed would be empty. I tried to stay in that moment with him by twirling his hair around my fingers, continuing to match his breathing with mine.

This was my prayer, "Dear God, please wrap your Angels wings around Joe, please heal him and give him peace. Please give me patience and the strength to handle this disease; please don't let Joe suffer!"

four

"Worry, worry every day, it can take your breath away."
Wanda

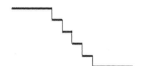

oe's son, Matt lived with Raechael, a wonderful woman he met in high school; they lived in Minnesota. Because of logistics, we did not see them often. Instead, we would visit on the phone. Joe loved his son and Raechael and sorely missed them. I had not told them that Joe was sick, because I did not want to worry them until I had a firm diagnosis. Now, I could put off this phone call no longer. I struggled for two days trying to work up the courage. I could not find the words.

It was a beautiful, sunny morning. I was lulled into a false sense of peace as I sat on our patio watching Joe wander through his rose garden. He was wearing his Tilley hat, which my mom had given him right after we moved into our home. He donned blue jeans, white tennis shoes and a navy blue long sleeve t-shirt and brown leather gloves. Whistling, he lovingly wandered through his roses as he pulled the occasional errant weed. Riley our Scottish terrier danced at his feet.

I snapped out of my quiet revere and dialed Matt and Raechaels number, my heart was beating so fast I could barely speak as Raechael answered the phone.

"Hello!"

"Hi, Raechael, it is Wanda."

"How are you?" she asked.

"Not good, Raechael."

"I have something to tell you." I paused, took a deep breath and said, "Joe is sick, he's been having memory problems for a while, but I didn't want to call you until I knew what it was. I don't know how to say this; Joe has Alzheimer's."

I blurted this out in the worst way possible; I had no experience in delivering this kind of news. Raechael was so stunned that for a moment I could not hear her breathing.

Finally, I asked, "Are you still there?"

"Yes." She said in a very quiet voice.

I could hear the beginnings of a sob as she said; "I'll get Matt, hang on."

It took a few moments for Matt to come on the line; he was very quiet as I told him what had been happening to his dad. Matt wanted to know everything, I told him the prognosis as he listened intently.

"Matt, I really think you and Raechael should come and see your dad. I don't know how much longer he'll know you. If it's possible, please come soon. Joe and I need you."

"Ok, Wanda, I'll call the airlines and we'll come as soon as possible. I'll call you back when I book our flight. I'm so sorry Wanda this is horrible news. How's my dad now?"

"Matt, your dad has never been happier; he's working in his roses, playing with Riley. He's eating and sleeping great. I actually have never seen him so peaceful and happy."

"I'm glad for that, I'll see you soon, oh Wanda, thank you for taking such good care of my dad."

"Don't thank me, I love him so much, Matt." I started to cry as I hung up the phone.

Joe came up to me and cuddled saying, "Don't cry, my love, everything is alright!"

It felt so good to be in his arms, I loved this man so much. Joe was right, now at this very moment everything was all right. I just could not look forward or backward. I was in the moment with him now, his strong body wrapped tightly around me, kept me there safe for now.

Joe was in a good place, having Alzheimer's, while becoming a challenge in day-to-day life had afforded some unexpected benefits. Before, Joe had been very Midwestern stuffy. Now, he had lost some of his inhibitions and had become more relaxed, lighthearted, and downright funny. He liked to play and he laughed a lot more.

In order to stay in his world, I had to become more like him, so I taught myself to stay with him in his present moment. Alzheimer's patients can only see the present moment, they live in the now. This kept me enjoying the little things and when I would start to worry, he would snap me out of my mood with a child-like smile or a hug. Stay in the moment, stay in the moment I told myself repeatedly. Focus on what is happening now, do not look back and do not look forward. Concentrate on how you feel now; this attitude became my way of life. Matching his mood to mine became my pleasure and daily goal.

I was so relieved that I had called his children, now I could relax and eagerly await their arrival. After a hearty meal of pasta and salad, Joe and I snuggled up with Riley on the couch to watch a movie. Joe fell asleep as I watched him, memorizing his face. My mind wandered back to the day he moved in with me and the two-week road trip we took across the country.

five

JANUARY 1998

*J*oe and I spent every day together since our meeting at Christmas. One morning, Joe arrived at my little trailer early, just after first light. We had coffee on the front steps. It was so romantic talking in quiet, hushed voices about our future, the rest of the trailer park was still sleeping. My White Knight took my hand in his and began stroking the inside of my right wrist with his thumb.

I felt weak with anticipation as he gazed lovingly into my eyes and said, "Wanda, I love you, I think it's time we moved in together, what do you think."

I could not think while he was stroking my wrist, he caught me off guard and I hesitated. Joe took that opportunity to lean into me and kiss me gently on the lips. I melted into him, receiving his kiss with eager lips.

I finally pulled away flushed and with barely a whisper said, "Yes, yes move in with me. I love you too."

Our time together was glorious. I was living a romance novel. Joe was my White Knight in Shining Armor.

At the end of February, Joe decided he had to go back to Iowa to finish a remodel project he had started for one of his friends. He would be gone for almost two months; I was devastated. I cried every day, I could not sleep at night and at work, I was a disaster. I did not think I would ever see him again.

About a week after he left, Joe started calling me at night. We would spend hours on the phone; he started writing me love letters, sending me little gifts, mostly jewelry. I also started writing him poems. This was my favorite:

MY LOVING MATE

When we were young, you took my hand
And walked into our future.
I gazed into your loving eyes and promises were made.
We stood together side by side, as life rolled all around us.
Our love was strong; some days were long,
But, through it all our love stood tall!
The days are slower; shoulders seem a little slumped.
Tired eyes not a light with wonder.
Come take my hand, my loving mate and walk into our future.
I gaze into your loving eyes and promises are made.
We'll stand together side by side, as life rolls all around us.
Our love is strong; some days are long,
But, through it all our love stands tall.
Our days are done upon this earth,
The winds have all blown by us.
Come take my hand, my loving mate and gaze into our future.
You are my one and only love, you'll walk with me forever.
Wanda

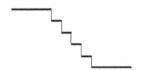

Six weeks after Joe left, he called one evening to say he was sending me a one-way ticket to Nebraska. We would drive up to Minnesota to see his kids, then a slow leisurely two-week road trip home to California. Joe was driving back his old van and all of his tools. I was flabbergasted; the farthest I had ever traveled was Texas. I got so excited I almost forgot I was afraid to fly!

My flight from California to Nebraska was exciting to say the least. I had called my Doctor and got a small prescription of Valium. I was so scared to fly; I thought that they would help take the edge off. They did not work.

Instead, I enlisted the cooperation of the handsome businessman seated next to me on the plane. Taking a deep breath, I began to engage him in meaningless conversation. At first, he tried to ignore me but upon realizing that I was not going away, he reluctantly closed his laptop and began to answer my questions. We spent the rest of the flight getting to know each other. He was very sweet and attentive and very disappointed that as we landed I quickly told him I was meeting Joe, the man of my dreams. With a wry smile and a quick hug, he disappeared from my life.

Joe was an hour late picking me up at the airport; I began to worry that he was not coming. Then all of a sudden, he burst through the double doors, threw his hands in the air and ran to me. He was dressed in dark blue jeans, white tennis shoes and a green and white parka. As he rushed up to me, I held my breath accepting his warm embrace. My body, now limp in his arms, was his forever.

Still weak from our embrace, Joe steered me out to his red van. I stood there speechless, it was very old most of the paint was either faded or rusted. There were a few dents and many scratches; the driver's side windshield had a large crack. This beloved van had seen better days. Joe threw open the side door to reveal a built in double bed complete with a brass headboard. He even had a bedspread tucked neatly under the mattress.

"Well, what do you think, I know it's old, but it will get us home." He proudly professed.

I started laughing and said, "It's unbelievable, I love the bed, I think the headboard is the most romantic touch!"

"Nothing is too good for you, my love. Hop in we have a four-hour drive to Iowa, we are meeting a friend of mine for dinner. Sorry I was late; traffic was bad leaving the city. Oh, by the way put your purse in the back some of the floorboards are missing in front, you don't want it falling in the highway!"

"Okay," I laughed hopping into the front seat.

I was awestruck at the landscape, which stretched ahead of us in flat manicured splendor. Either side of the four-lane highway was planted in lawn that stretched from Nebraska to Iowa. For four hours, I waited to see the man responsible for mowing this lush green grass.

It was fun having dinner with Joe's friend. We had lively conversation and good home-cooked food. Joe and I went back to his friend's house alone and spent the night in loving passion. I was so far out of my comfort zone, and yet felt very much at home with Joe. He was solid, like a rock, my loving White Knight.

Waking up next to Joe the next morning was so exciting, he rolled over and pulled me into his arms, we laid there not speaking for what seemed like forever, when all of a sudden he jumped out of bed and said, "Get up the days a wasting! We're driving to Minneapolis today to see my kids, hurry I am hungry, we'll go out to breakfast and head out!"

I laughed; he was always ready to eat! "Ok, let's go, I'm hungry too, but I'm nervous to meet your children!"

Joe always referred to Raechael as one of his "children." He had known her since she was in high school and started dating Matt.

"Oh, don't worry; they're going to love you as much as I do!"

We had a hearty breakfast then back in Joe's old red van and headed for Minneapolis. The countryside was breathtaking; everywhere I looked was blue sky and lush green vegetation. It took us a few hours to get to our destination. We were so busy talking I did not feel the time pass, being with Joe was timeless. He was so relaxed and easy going that I relaxed just being with him.

Matt, and Raechael met us outside as we pulled into their driveway. Joe jumped out of his van and was in their arms before I could get out of the van. I gingerly walked up to them and was welcomed with hugs.

"This is Wanda, the love of my life." Joe said proudly.

"We know who she is Dad, come in, are you hungry?" They chimed in at once.

Dinner was delicious, steak, vegetables and salad. Matt and Raechael had been together since high school. It was so much fun to get to know the two people that Joe loved most on this earth. Raechael was independent, strong and bubbled with personality. Matt was so like Joe, quiet with a quick sense of humor, very intelligent and sensitive. You could tell how much he loved Raechael; they kept eye contact even when engaged in conversation. I fell instantly in love with Joe's children. They had a beautiful presence about them and made me feel very welcome.

"We made up the guest room for you tonight." Matt said.

"No, thank you we'll stay in the van. I built us a bed; we would rather not put you out. We're leaving at first light tomorrow headed back for California." Joe responded.

"Can we at least make you breakfast in the morning?" Rachael asked.

"We'll eat on the road; you'll still be in bed when we leave." Joe said.

Because we only had one day with them we stayed up very late to squeeze in every moment. On the way to the van, I asked Joe why he was in such a hurry to leave.

"I love my children, but I am anxious to start our road trip, I want everything from now on to be about us. I'm sorry if that sounds selfish, but when it comes to time with you, I guess I'm a little selfish."

"Yes, you are, but I love you and I'm also excited to get started."

With that, we curled around each other and fell fast asleep, with the promise of a lifetime of tomorrows in our dreams.

Joe woke me at first light by lightly kissing my hand, then my arm slowly working his way to my lips. What followed was sweet, poignant passion ending in an explosion of love so intense that I had to gulp for air. Then the familiar tears, again he touched my soul.

We quickly dressed and drove off to a hearty breakfast and our bright future.

South Dakota was the first time Joe had a lapse in memory on our trip. We stopped at K-mart to buy a few things we needed for the trip and Joe locked the keys in the van. We spent the next hour with Joe using a wire coat hanger threading it through one of many holes in the side of the van to unlock the door. I laughed so hard I had to run back into K-mart to use the bathroom. When someone locks the keys in a car who suspects a problem? Everyone does that; right?

The next leg of our trip took us over the Continental Divide, during a snowstorm. I immediately panicked.

"Pull over Joe, until the storm passes!"

"I can't do that, if we pull over now, we'll be here for days and we'll probably freeze to death!" he calmly declared.

"I'm scared we're going to slip off this mountain." I yelled back.

"We're ok, remember, I've spent the last twenty years in Minnesota, I'm comfortable driving in the snow."

"Oh, yeah, I forgot."

I held on for dear life as Joe carefully guided us down that angry mountain and when we reached the bottom, I looked over at him, sweat pouring off my brow and said. "That wasn't so bad!"

He turned to look at me and laughed.

Twenty minutes later we pulled into a gas station, the truck needed gas and Joe needed coffee and a doughnut.

I threw open the truck door very happy to put my feet on solid ground and the fierce winds almost took the door off. We were out in the middle of nowhere.

I yelled above the gale. "I'm going inside to use the bathroom."

"Ok, I will be in after I get gas." He yelled back.

Once inside the small convenience store, I felt better until I looked around. The man behind the counter had to be at least six feet tall, with thick shaggy long black hair. His beard hit the middle of his very round belly. When he smiled at me, he had two missing front teeth. There was another man off towards the back of the store that looked just like him.

"Which way to the bathroom?" I timidly asked.

"Down that aisle and to the right, little lady." He politely replied.

Joe felt far away, as I entered the bathroom. My mouth fell open as I looked around; it was a very large room, with white dingy walls. Sitting side by side were two toilets. I looked behind me to lock the door, much to my surprise, no lock. I had no choice but to use one of the toilets. I wondered if two people would use both toilets at the same time. I was very far from home indeed!

I met Joe at the counter as he was paying for gas and two cups of stale coffee and two doughnuts.

I ran back to the van, but not before looking around. There behind the store was an old school bus, deserted and beat up.

As I closed the door, I said to Joe, "Where have all the children gone? I bet that guy behind the counter is the Mayor and Police Chief." We both laughed.

Joe and I continued on our journey that day and ended up in Cody, Wyoming a small town a few hours away. Its main street was a two-lane road. Joe's truck had many problems one of which was chugging; it ran great at 45 miles an hour not so great at 10 miles an hour. We were so busy trying to get his truck to the campsite that we failed to notice that the van was filling up with smoke. However, the local police noticed a fire under the van. Next thing we knew they pulled us over, Joe thought we were getting a ticket for going too fast! The police officer stopped us, and opened the van door ordering us out, Joe tried to argue, and the police officer almost yanked him out of our van.

Joe yelled, "Grab my wallet and your purse, we're on fire!"

"What?" I snapped back.

"Get out of the van, it's on fire!" He shouted.

I rushed to obey him and got out, my heart pounding. The police officer stopped our van in front of a church so we sat on the steps to watch the show. Every firefighter in the small city and two fire trucks came towards us sirens screaming! Six Firemen jumped out of their trucks, unraveling miles of hose to put out our fire. In the meantime, the police chief and the fire chief were arguing about a fire that no one could now see! It was the funniest thing I had ever seen. Joe and I sat there trying not to laugh, our cheeks hurt from holding back the laughter.

The fire chief finally told us to go on ahead a couple of blocks to the local car wash, and hose off the underneath of the van, we smiled and said ok! The van barely ran as we chugged down the next two blocks laughing! When we got to the car wash, I jumped out to get some quarters, I handed them to Joe.

He said in a very serious voice, "You'd better stand back, when I hit this van with the water, parts of her are going to spray all over this parking lot!"

"You're kidding me!" I laughed.

"No, I'm not! Get behind that wall" He laughed back.

I did not believe him, as soon as he started the water there was a swirling of metal parts, which looked like a small tornado. I could not contain myself, I laughed so hard I almost lost it. I ended up squatting on the ground not able to breathe.

Joe looked over at me so serious and said, "Told you!"

He did not let it faze him; he acted as if this was just another normal day at the car wash, which made the whole experience even funnier!

After the car wash the van was so wet it would not start, Joe had to climb underneath the van to hook up some wires that had come loose. I ran across the street to buy food to barbeque. I kept waiting for him to explode, the day had been one mishap after another, but Joe stayed amazingly calm. When I got back, Joe was in the van happy as a clam and all wet!

The van chugged two more blocks to the campground, which was empty. Joe went into the office to pay, and I picked our camp-site and set up the tent. We were so busy we failed to notice the sky filling up with very dark, low very forbidding clouds. Just as our steaks were coming off the grill, we heard the first clap of thunder. It was so close that you could feel it in your chest.

Joe yelled," Hurry, we have to get all this stuff in the van!"

I yelled back, "OK!"

We took down the tent, put our food on paper plates and headed for the van. No sooner did we shut the doors, than it began to rain, thunder and lightning lit up the evening sky. I had never before seen such a wild storm. We started laughing and ate our dinner, then headed back to our double bed. We laid there all night in that cozy, old van and listened to the most beautiful music God has ever put on this earth, the sound of new life, the sound of rain.

We did not make love; instead, we snuggled and held each other, waking up at first light still in each other's arms. Staying in the moment was easy with Joe in our early days; he commanded my attention with his intense love of me.

The highlight of our trip was camping in the Black Hills. It was the end of April and we were the only people camping. Joe and I picked out a beautiful campsite near the river. After we settled in and prepared a fabulous dinner, we spent the evening snuggling and watching the stars come out in a blanket of light that hovered reverently just above our heads.

We made passionate love that night in our warm and cozy tent, no one to hear us but the wildlife!

About three in the morning, I got up to use the bathroom, which was up a hill about 500 yards away. Joe heard me and quickly got up to escort me.

"No, stay in bed, I can go by myself."

"No way, you don't know what's out there; I'll feel better if I go with you."

"OK, I'm sorry I woke you."

"That's ok; I don't want you out of my sight!"

"Put your coat on, it's cold out."

I donned my coat and shoes and we headed to the bathroom. The night was so clear that the stars pressed down on us. On our way, back we could hear the distance howling of coyotes and I could hear the brush near us rustling, I grabbed Joe's arm.

Suddenly we both stopped in our tracks, above us and to the left the sky erupted in billowy ribbons of pastel light. Undulating with the rhythm of nature, the lights danced above and around us. I was too shocked to speak. Joe was silent.

"What's that?" I whispered.

"The Northern Lights." Joe reverently replied.

"Oh, my God, it's so beautiful!"

We sat down where we stood and holding each other close watched as Mother Nature displayed her grandeur. It was a "holy" moment, we did not speak; each lost in our own thoughts.

The next morning Joe was up early and had started a fire and put on the coffee. I started to climb out of the tent as he stopped me.

"Wanda, it's really cold, here, put on my down gloves and coat, you might freeze!"

"I'll be ok, I'm tough."

"Not that tough, don't argue with me."

I obeyed and gratefully accepted his coat as I stood up and looked around. Everything was white, it had snowed during the night and the temperature was in the twenties.

"Ohhh! mmmy GGGod!" I said as I tried to speak, my lips were numb and the air was so cold, that it left me breathless.

While we huddled near the fire, Joe began to rub my arms and legs. "Don't worry, once the sun comes over that mountain, the snow will melt."

"Whh Whh When will that happen?" I shivered.

"About eleven!" Then he laughed.

I would have laughed, but I could not move my lips.

We quickly drank our coffee, ate a meager breakfast and headed for town, grateful for the luxurious heat of the van.

Joe and I camped in the Black Hills for four days, touring the Indian reservations before heading for California thru Utah and the most beautiful scenery I have ever seen. We stopped many times just to take in the magnificent vistas before us. I tried to capture on film what I was experiencing, but would always stop, it seemed like an insult somehow.

When we finally arrived in Reno, Nevada, we stopped in a casino parking lot and went into dinner. We enjoyed a wonderful meal of steak, baked potatoes and we shared chocolate cake for desert. We went dancing and Joe matched my passion moving with me slowly and passionately to the music; we were born to dance together!

six

First Light

Have I talked about my search, for "first light"?
That moment between darkness and the dawn of a new day.
We need to pursue that time together for the rest of our lives.
I think that "first light" is in the heart and the soul.
That time together between birth and death.

Wanda

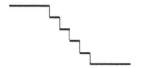

JUNE 2005

J woke up to the news on the television, "Oh no!" we slept on the couch all night. I stiffly hobbled to the bathroom. I really had to stop thinking about the past. The corners of my mouth tipped up as I remembered our road trip, the trip of a lifetime, a lifetime ago.

I was startled out of my reverie by Joe as he asked, "What's for breakfast?"

"I'll meet you in the kitchen, give me a moment."

"Back to reality and the start of a new day, stay in the moment Wanda, stay in the moment." I whispered to myself.

I reminded myself of how easy I had stayed in the moment with Joe on our trip. I took a deep breath, centered myself, and watched as I splashed cold water on my face, the way it felt, the sound of my breath. I brought myself back to the moment and did not anticipate the future.

Joe was in a great mood this morning. He kept giving me the look; you know the look a lover gives his partner when they have a shared secret. It was as if he had traveled back with me last night to our romantic cross-country trip. No, that was not possible; then again, it did seem very real!

Thank God, it was Saturday, today we were demolishing the guest bathroom. Matt and Raechael would be here in a few weeks and our bathroom was a disaster. They had never been to our house and I wanted it to look cozy for them. I tore out the toilet, sink and flooring. Then I would paint. My son in law, Brady said he would install the new flooring and the sink and toilet.

Joe could not do any remodeling on his own, but was anxious to help me. With a quick grin, he launched into helping, which mostly meant watching me. He could still follow directions and could hand me things; we had a fun and productive day. By nightfall our bathroom was empty, tomorrow we would paint. I realized I had stayed in the moment with Joe all day.

We fell into bed exhausted, before I could adjust my pillow Joe was sleeping. I laid there watching television mindlessly flipping through the channels. My mind wandered back to our wedding and my dad's death.

JUNE 1998

We were rough housing in our little trailer that I had rented before we met, when Joe suddenly tossed me on the bed, fell on top of me, looked me in the eyes and in a very passionate voice said, "Wanda, I love you! Will you marry me?"

I stopped; I could not believe what I had just heard.

"Yes!" I said.

Then, I said, "Ask me again!"

"Wanda, I love you will you be my wife?"

"Yes!"

He kissed me tenderly, we pulled apart and I said, "Ask me again!"

"Well, maybe I should think about it." He said laughing.

"One more time, please, I don't ever want to forget this moment!" I whispered.

"Will you please, please marry me? I love you and want to spend the rest of my life with you."

"Well, if you are going to be so insistent about it, ok!"

Then we made love, long and slow.

Joe was very absent-minded! He lost his wallet 3 times before our wedding! Each time someone would call with his wallet, I bought a cake to say thank you. The last time was two days before we were to get our marriage license; I was upset.

When the nice man that found it, called us I told Joe, "I am going to keep your wallet in my purse until after we get married. If this keeps up I'm going to tie your wallet around your neck, this is getting expensive; three cakes in as many months!"

We both laughed and went about preparing another great dinner. People lost things all the time; why should I worry!

We planned our Wedding for Friday August 7, 1998. Our plans changed suddenly as my father, who had been battling prostate cancer died.

I had gone to work early that day; Joe and I were getting married at one that afternoon. Cheryl had bought us a cake and she had bought me flowers for a bouquet.

I worked in Hayward and it was usually about a two-hour drive.

I had barely put down my purse when the phone rang and my sister Trudy said, "Wanda, come home dad is back in the hospital, he's dying. They'll try to wait until you get here so you can say good-bye before they administer morphine."

"What? I'll come back as fast as I can, but it's rush hour, it will probably take me three hours to get back to Watsonville. If he's in pain, don't wait, give him the morphine!"

I grabbed my purse as I ran to my bosses' office and in a breathless voice; as I gulped for air, told him about my dad. He came from behind his desk and hugged me and I began to cry.

"Wanda, take all the time you need, but be careful driving, you're upset and I'm worried. Do you want me to drive you home?"

"No, I'll be ok, the traffic is crawling, and the hardest part will be thinking about him and not being there. I'll call you later today, the company picnic is tomorrow, I know I'm in charge, I left everything I had to bring on my desk, I'm so sorry!"

With that, I flew out to my car to begin the long, slow ride home. I was in a daze; my dad was dying. Other people had their dads die, but my dad, never! I could not imagine my life without him. I always felt so strong knowing he was there for me. My poor mom, I could not put myself in her place. Her husband of forty-six years was leaving her; he was going home.

I remembered the day Joe and I cut down his last new Town Pippin apple tree. Dad had had a five-way bypass surgery and was still recovering. His last apple tree was dying and needed to be cut down. Joe offered to do it for him and my dad readily agreed.

Joe and I arrived at my parent's farm early on a Saturday morning and after a short visit, we began the sad and arduous task of bringing down his last tree. We lived on six acres of apples. Six months before my dad had pulled out all of his New Town Pippin trees. They were at least one hundred years old and replaced them with sixteen hundred Fuji apple trees. My dad was so proud of his new orchard!

Joe started the chain saw and just before he made the first cut I yelled, "Stop! Before you cut her down, can I have a picture of me with her?"

Joe turned off the saw and said, "Yes, that's a good idea, let me get my camera."

I climbed up into the old tree as I had done a hundred times before as a young girl for her last picture. A treasured picture proudly displayed in my bedroom.

I slammed on my breaks as the driver in front of me merged into my lane. I began to pray for my dad, "Please God don't let my dad suffer today, take him into your loving arms, peacefully. Please God, let me get there to say good-by before he goes."

I wiped away tears as I pulled into the hospital parking lot.

My family greeted me at the hospital, they were sober and quiet; my mom was in with my dad.

"Go in and say good-bye, we already did. We're sorry they just administered the morphine. I don't think he'll know you're there." Trudy, my sister said.

I hugged each of them, took a deep breath and pushed open the door to his room.

My mom was sitting next to my dad holding his hand. I stood there, not moving, mom came and put her arms around me.

"Oh, my God, mom is dad really dying?"

"Yes, Wanda, it's his time. I'll go out so you can say good-by."

After she left, I gingerly walked around the bed, sat down and picked up his hand.

"Dad, it's Wanda, I love you. You've been the best dad in the world. Can you feel my hand, dad?"

He gently squeezed my hand, his eyes closed. I continued, "Its ok for you to go now, go, daddy and fly with the angels. Mom will be all right. We're all here, we'll take good care of her, don't worry."

"Please God; take good care of my dad!" I silently prayed.

I sat there and watched him breathe. My life with this incredible man flashed before me. I knew I would never again here his jolly voice as he would hug me and say, "Hi daughter, how are you? What do you think?"

"Think about what, dad, give me a topic." Then we would both laugh and he would hug me tighter.

There were no words, only silent flashes of love and comfort. My heart was racing and he was with me. I could feel him feel me. Tears stung my eyes as I watched my dad struggle to breathe. Finally, I could not stand another minute, I leaned over stroked his forehead, kissed him gently and said, "Goodbye daddy, we'll meet again." Then, I walked out to be with my family.

He passed away early Saturday morning August 8. His funeral was the following Saturday and so large that we had to have the reception at the hall, next to the church. He was loved and respected; I missed him dearly.

Joe and I were married in a small ceremony, Wednesday August 19. It was bittersweet, happy because I was marrying Joe, sad because I ached for my dad. It was the first big event of my life that he missed. We did not go on a honeymoon, promising ourselves that when things calmed down we would go, we never did.

seven

"I was witness today to the miracle of love, a very old couple sat in a
convalescent hospital holding hands and snuggling with each other.
They had been married for over fifty years. I stood captivated by their
feelings for each other after all those years. I thought of us. I thought of our
children and how love knows no bounds, no age and has no boundaries."

Joe

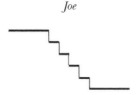

JULY 2005

Joe woke me up with a head bump; I laid there remembering my dad and our wedding. Joe was asking for food as
I remembered it was painting day. I wiped tears from my eyes.

"Get up Wanda, it's a new day." I said to myself as I headed for
the bathroom. "Stay in the moment, stay in the moment."

This time to stay in the moment I focused on Joe, his smiling
and happy face, the way he gently stroked my arm, while gingerly
pulling me out of my warm cozy bed.

I painted all day, while Joe watched. He spent most of his
time in his rose garden, picking weeds and playing with Riley. By
nightfall, I was stiff and exhausted.

Brady completed our bathroom just a week before Matt and Raechael arrived. It was with nervous anticipation that I awaited their arrival. I had only met them once and was unsure of their reaction to Joe's illness. I also was not sure, how Joe would react and if he would remember them.

My fears were unfounded as Joe bounded out of the car in the parking lot and rushed up to his children. He scooped each one into his loving arms for a long hug. My heart swelled with pride as I watched this loving exchange. Matt and Raechael were beautiful, articulate and loving children, I breathed a sigh of relief; this reunion was going to be just what they all needed.

After a long, slow breakfast, with spirited and lively banter and much reminiscing, we headed back to Jim and Cheryl's house. We spent the rest of the day laughing and loving Joe's children. I could not have loved them more if I had given birth to them myself. I counted the moments that day, each one precious.

Jim was so proud of Matt and Raechael; I gave Jim time to spend alone with them so he could talk about Joe. After another one of Cheryl's fabulous meals, we headed back to our home and much needed sleep. We were all exhausted.

I put Joe to bed and finally had a chance to talk to Matt and Raechael alone. They asked many questions, which I tried to answer in an honest and gentle manner. As I talked about Joe, I began to cry, Raechael cried too.

"How is my dad, really?" Matt asked refusing to cry.

"Your dad is very happy; he is unraveling, like a baby grows. Joe is becoming less inhibited and very funny; he is more relaxed and less stiff. He doesn't seem to realize that anything is wrong."

"How much time does my dad have, how long will this last?" Matt queried in a serious deep voice.

"Well, originally, his doctor said two years, but I have put him on a drug, which will not cure him but extend the quality of his life. How long, I'm not sure."

Matt lowered his head, fighting back unshed tears. My heart broke for this strong, young man.

Raechael, the most pragmatic of the two asked, "What can we do for Joe, what can we do for you?"

"Well, nothing, logistics are impossible. You live too far away to help day to day. The best thing you can do for your dad and me is to call often. I want Joe to remember you for as long as possible. If he can hear your voices, I think that will help. Also pray for your dad, pray for all of us." I had to clear my throat as I was having trouble talking and not crying.

Raechael said, "We will come back to visit again, often."

"Yes, we'll come back again, soon." Matt reiterated.

We hugged each other and I basked in their love, I was so in love with them. I could hear their hearts breaking and I could do nothing to stop it. I felt powerless. A restless sadness seeped into the rest of their trip. They were new to California and there was much to see. They both carved out time to spend alone with their dad. Joe's carefree attitude stood in stark contrast to the sadness felt by his children.

The morning of their departure was hectic. We took many pictures and promised each other to get together soon. The last hugs delivered, and the last tears shed, Matt and Raechael piled into their rental car and drove away. I stood in our front yard holding Joe, waving good-by and wondering if Joe would ever really "see" them again, or would they be familiar strangers next time.

Joe walked back in the house and asked for food, our last few days with his beloved children gone from his memory. However, I hoped embedded in his soul forever.

That night sleep would not come, my mind played back the kids visit and how happy and relieved I was that Joe had gotten to once again, spend time with them. I was starring death in the face and all I could see was my past with Joe. We had lived a rich life in a short time. Joe and I had not wasted one day, not one moment. I did not sleep that night as I relived our amazing story.

OCTOBER 1998

After getting married, our little trailer seemed too small and we began to look for a house, somewhere in Scott's valley, we loved it there. With very little effort, we found an enchanting little cottage in the woods in Ben Lomond on Huckleberry Island, surrounded by the San Lorenzo River. There were twenty houses built in the last century, our cabin was originally a caretakers cottage for the main house. It was for rent and without even seeing the inside; we took it.

The property was beautiful; our cabin hidden under a thick canopy of redwoods was only one hundred yards from the river. There were two stands of trees, one outside our front door and one outside our kitchen window. Enchanted was the only word for our new world in the mountains. This was home to me, I felt like I was born to live there. This was where peace and love was born for me.

We stood open-mouthed as we entered our little cabin for the first time. There was no kitchen, only an empty room with a refrigerator in the hallway. There were three small bedrooms, the master was an add-on, and had a bathroom sink in the wall. The outside window was still there overlooking the living room from the master. The only little bathroom had a claw foot bathtub and a window that looked out onto the laundry room. Overall, it was a mélange of chaos, but adorable to us. The walls to our cabin were one-inch redwood, filled with many holes that you could actually see through. The cabin sported a floor furnace in the living room, it's only source of heat. There were original hardwood floors in terrible disrepair. French doors hung in regal beauty for the front and back doors.

Our landlord handed us our keys looking embarrassed as he noted our expressions. He ran his hand through his thick white hair, shaking his head.

Joe shook his hand and in an excited voice said, "I can remodel this, I will add a kitchen, if that's all right with you!"

"Thank you, do anything you want, make it your own. I am so grateful to have you and your wife as tenants."

Joe ran to his truck, got his measuring tape, and began to envisage and measure our new home for a working kitchen.

"Don't worry, Wanda, this will be the most beautiful home we've ever had."

I grabbed him, took his face in my hands, and said, "I know Joe, I know, I trust you, it'll be fun to work on our new little home together."

Joe ran back to his truck, grabbed a blanket, threw it on the master bedroom floor and made passionate love to me. Then, we happily headed off to the lumberyard to gather supplies to begin our remodel.

There are times in a person's life that stand out as stellar. That was how that year in our little care takers cottage was for us. With all of our senses heightened, we spent every waking moment working on our home. We both had to work in the daytime, me in Hayward, which was a two-hour commute each way and Joe worked for the local union. Every night and all weekend, we continued to build our little home from the inside out.

Finally, after six months of blood, sweat and yes, a few tears, our home was finished. White cabinets with navy blue knobs sat proudly on a navy blue and white tile floor. Navy Formica graced our new wrap around counter top.

The pained windows throughout the house were dressed with white Pricilla curtains. We painted the inside of our home white, which stood in stark contrast to the dark green woods. Joe removed the bathroom sink in our bedroom and added a much-needed closet. Our biggest and most prized possession was a 1900 four-poster cannonball bed that dominated our bedroom. We painted the bathroom white and Joe added a shower in our antique claw foot tub.

Our cabin became our home and as charming and filled with love as we were. We celebrated by having a house warming party. All of our family and friends came to welcome us home.

Joe began having trouble getting regular work with the union. He worked very slow and was so methodical that he could not keep pace with the rest of the crew. I was beginning to have trouble paying our bills. I was the only one working.

A friend of ours had moved to Las Vegas and loved it, while I was voicing my concerns to her one day she said, "Wanda, why don't you and Joe move here, there is lots of work and I am sure I can get you both jobs with my company. It would be great to have you guys here with me, I miss you and Joe."

"Vegas! I don't know, it's so hot there. I don't know if I can leave my job, I've been there for thirteen years."

"Wanda, start over, as long as you are with Joe, who cares where you live. Think outside the box and take a chance. I did and I love it here. Please, just think about it. I will call you tomorrow, talk to Joe, it's a good idea. I love you."

eight

"Being in the right place at the right time is an act of God,
wherever you are is where you are supposed to be. Never question that,
always know for certain, listen to your heart and watch the signs!"

Joe

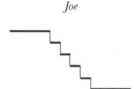

JANUARY 1999

The balance of our year was relatively uneventful, although I was still having trouble paying bills. We decided to put off moving for a while and it turned out to be a good call. Then, in January, we had a crisis with Jim. Cheryl had been telling me that Jim was having trouble with his stomach.

One afternoon she called me and said, "Wanda, come quick, Jim is in terrible pain!"

I responded, "We will be right there!"

Joe and I flew to Jim and Cheryl's house just as the ambulance was pulling up. The paramedics gingerly placed Jim on a stretcher, his face twisted in pain; he was barely able to speak. They loaded him in the ambulance and Joe and I followed with Cheryl to the hospital.

In the emergency room, the doctors could not diagnose Jim. Joe was very upset and paced nervously about his room. One of the emergency doctors asked us if Jim had had any previous problems with his stomach.

Joe said, "No, but it reminds me of the problems I had with my stomach."

The doctor was quick to react, "What problems did you have?"

Joe said, "I had my intestines rupture about 10 years ago, no one could figure out what was wrong, I almost died!"

Jim's doctor said because they were twins, they could have inherited the same problems with their intestines. They did a scan of Jim's stomach and he was in surgery within an hour.

Thank God Joe was there that day and knew enough to tell the doctor about himself. I believe that day we saw a miracle, if they had delayed even an extra hour, Jim could have died. Jim had a colostomy for a couple of months, which he hated. He was not a very patient, patient! Joe spent a lot of time with Jim while he was sick; they became inseparable.

Jim had his colostomy reversed in May and by August was again in trouble. This time it was with severe back pain; so bad that he could not work. His doctor finally sent him to a large hospital in the bay area for a second opinion. After the doctor there examined him, he said that Jim could not leave the office to drive home; his pain was coming from the vertebrae in his neck. His condition was so severe he risked paralysis simply by stepping off a curb! He needed surgery immediately. Jim was naturally upset and filled with disbelief; he thought himself to be invincible. Jim told the doctor he needed to go for a walk and call his wife.

The doctor warned," Be careful Jim!"

Jim called Cheryl; he needed her and she needed to pick up Palmer as he had taken him to the hospital that day. Cheryl filled with disbelief and in tears called me. She did not drive out of town and could not get to Jim or her dad.

"Wanda, Jim is at the hospital with my dad. His doctor said he needs immediate surgery, will you come home and take me to the hospital?"

I was at working in Hayward. As soon as I got the call, I went to my boss, told him of our family emergency; he gave me a week off with the sincere hope that everything would be ok. I drove home to Watsonville, which took about 2 hours. (We could not get ahold of Joe as he was out on a building site.)

Cheryl was pacing around the house in tears. Andon had left work to drive up to the hospital with us so he could drive Jim's truck home. He was beside himself with worry over his dad. Andon has always been a huge comfort to Cheryl and Jim. He was their only son. We jumped in the car and drove back to the bay area, another 2 hours, to be with Jim and to pick up Palmer.

They admitted Jim to the hospital by the time we got there. Palmer faithfully sat in a chair by his side. Palmer was very scared and upset; he seemed a little out of it and looked very pale. Andon and I gave Jim and Cheryl some privacy; we took Palmer out of the room. The atmosphere was thick with worry.

We said our good-byes for the night and Palmer padded quietly beside us out to the parking lot. He usually was very animated, but after his ordeal that day, we did not question his silence. Andon went to get Jim's truck in the parking garage and Cheryl was on the phone to her office, telling them she would be out for the week.

Palmer was standing next to me, and I noticed that he was sweating and rubbing his chest.

"Palmer, are you all right?"

He whispered, "Yes, but my chest hurts."

I said tenderly," Palmer sit down on this bench and take slow, deep breaths, I'll be right back."

I walked over to Cheryl; she had just gotten off the phone with her work, and I said," Cheryl, I think Palmer is having a heart attack."

Cheryl looked at me in disbelief and said, "What!"

Andon showed up with the truck, Palmer refused to go back into the hospital; he seemed better and just wanted to go home. We decided to take him to his doctor in Watsonville. Andon left with Palmer, and Cheryl and I followed them in my car. All the way home, we sat in stunned silence, Jim, now maybe Palmer! What an awful day!

By the time we got to Watsonville, Palmer was fine and refused to go to the hospital. Andon drove him to his house. I took Cheryl home, she very tired and upset; she was going to bed. I went home to tell Joe about our horrific day. I too was exhausted and could not believe how the day had unfolded.

"Joey, what if Jim comes out of this surgery and can't walk, what will Cheryl do? How can we help them?"

"Well, if that happens, we will move in with them and we will all help take care of Jim. We will take turns working. He is my brother and I will always take care of him and Cheryl." He said passionately pacing the kitchen.

"Thank God, that's what I was going to say, we're a family, we'll always take care of each other."

Palmer started feeling bad about 11pm that night, and drove himself to the hospital. The hospital called Cheryl about 12am. She had taken a sleeping pill and could not get to the hospital that night. The nurse assured Cheryl that Palmer would be all right for the night, she would see him the next morning.

It took the hospital two days to gather all of the titanium needed to repair Jim's vertebrae. His surgery took six hours; it was long and complicated. Even though it had been a success, Jim would have a long, slow recovery, with no guarantee of future pain. We were so thankful and relieved and did not want to think about the future.

While Jim was in surgery, Cheryl got a call from our local hospital asking her to pick up her dad. Palmer was very anxious to go home. The doctors inserted a stint; Palmer really did not understand what had happened to him. He just wanted to go home. We had to make Palmer wait until we could see Jim in recovery.

The day had gotten so complicated. Jim, as soon as he woke up in recovery also wanted to go home. Now, that both of our patients seemed to be out of the woods, we took a deep breath and headed home, our hearts lighter and our future brighter.

Jim's recovery went surprisingly fast. He had a small limp and still experienced pain. At least he was not in a wheel chair, we were all very grateful! We thanked God for our two miracles!

nine

"I'm free, I'm free the past is gone, I don't know how,
but I'm free of the pain, the guilt, the anguish.
You did this, I did this, and we did this.
I've found the eighteen-year-old girl I once was.
I can see her, feel her, and hear her. I feel light as a feather.
My future with you looks like heaven."

Wanda

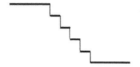

APRIL 2000

By April, Joe's work situation had become so tenuous that we had no choice but to take our friend's offer and move to Las Vegas. I would be an apartment manager for an apartment complex and Joe would be a maintenance manager. We would work together and live on site. Leaving our little cabin in the woods was fraught with anxiety. At least we could take Riley with us.

On our last day, with the last box packed, we walked down to our special place by the river hand in hand.

There by the water, Joe grabbed me for a full body hug, he whispered in my ear, "Wanda, I love you so much, I know how hard leaving your job and moving so far away from your family is on you. I know you are doing this for me. I love you for it and I will not let you down."

"I'm doing this for us, Joe, we are a team. Besides, I'm always up for a new adventure. Let's go Joey, let's start a new chapter in our lives. As long as we are together, it doesn't matter where we live."

With our last good-byes to our little cabin in the woods, we started out for Las Vegas and our future. I swallowed a lump in my throat, my heart felt heavy as I watched my hometown disappear from view.

Six months after we arrived in Vegas, Joe had another episode with memory loss. He set out to our near-by grocery store and was gone about twenty minutes. Joe suddenly rang our doorbell he did not use his key.

He stood in the door way and I asked," Joey, why are you here did you already go to the store?"

Joe said, "No, I got lost I couldn't find it, how do you get there again?"

I was very surprised, because Joe had been there many, many, times. I gave him directions and off he went. Later that night I asked him why he got lost and he said he did not know. I blew it off; after all, he was an old man of 52!

Our lives settled into a very comfortable routine, and the months just flew. We did not like Las Vegas but made the best of it. We were together so we danced, laughed, and delighted in our love. Even the desert has its own beauty, and we spent a lot of time with our new friends and sightseeing. We barbequed almost every night and took long walks with Riley.

I got a call from Joe's manager and the apartment manager; they wanted to have a meeting with me about Joe. I was weak with worry as I sat in their office. They said Joe was always getting lost on the property, which had about 300 units. When he would arrive at an apartment to answer a repair call, he would often not remember what he was supposed to fix, or forget his tools. They were letting him go; they called me in to say they thought he had memory problems.

"Maybe, he has Alzheimer's," they both said at once.

I was very angry. I sputtered as I said, "I have to carry a map of the units, so I don't get lost. This is a huge property. As far as forgetting tools, who hadn't done that?"

As I look back now, I realize I was making excuses for Joe's memory problems. However, at the time, I did not know anything about Alzheimer's and in every other way, he seemed so normal. We needed Joe to work to make ends meet, so he applied to a hardware store, and got the job! Of course, I just knew he was all right.

ten

"Have faith in me, my love.
Every day of my life with you is like the first day,
you continue to take my breath away"

Joe

JULY 2001 – APRIL 2004

ife calmed down, Joe did not like his new job, but went faithfully every day; they loved him there. About 6 months later, we decided to move back to Watsonville. I became increasingly uncomfortable about being so far away from Jim and Cheryl. A slowly budding fear always seemed just out of reach, hovering over my shoulder.

We moved in with Jim and Cheryl until we could find a house of our own. Joe transferred to the store in Gilroy, which was about thirty minutes away. I spent my days looking for a new job. It was such a relief to be home, it felt safe to be so near Jim. I was lulled into a false sense of security and began to relax. One evening after Joe had gone to bed, Jim came to me and wanted to talk.

"Have you noticed anything different about Joe?" He asked.

I answered puzzled, "No, he seems fine to me, they love him at work, why do you ask?"

Jim said," I don't know. He just seems different to me, oh, well maybe I'm imagining things."

We never brought the subject up to each other again. Jim was very protective of Joe and I never gave our conversation anymore thought until years later.

Joe and I found a house in a senior community in Watsonville to rent, it was very cozy, which means small with a large backyard! Joe and I immediately began to feather our nest. The first thing we did after we painted the inside of our house was to stain all the fencing in the backyard. For us, re-doing a house was entertainment. On the weekends, we would go antiquing; we both loved the hunt for the old and unique. Then we planted a rose garden.

For Joe's birthday I asked everyone to bring a bare root rose bush, Joe loved roses and could not grow them in Minnesota. I thought that would be a great gift. Joe was overwhelmed and proud of his thirty rose bushes. After we lovingly planted the roses, we planted vegetables. Our yard was beautiful! Joe spent every day in his garden, lovingly tending to his roses. I worked by his side in our vegetable garden, we were just like two old farmers. We worked by day and at night became sensuous, tender lovers.

We had many parties, and holidays in our cozy little home and we were very happy. Joe continued to do well at the hardware store. Towards the end of our third year in rental home, we started looking for a house to buy and found one just down the street in the same neighborhood.

Matt and Raechael were married June 8. Joe and I were thrilled. Raechael was already a part of our family and we loved her dearly. We lived too far away to go to their wedding but we were there in spirit. They sent us many beautiful pictures, which Joe proudly displayed in our living room.

Joe had hernia surgery in May, which was uneventful. Two weeks off work and he was ready to go back. He did not like having to lie around the house recuperating. We watched many movies during those two weeks, I spent most of my time telling him, "No, Joe don't lift that!"

The rest of the year and all of the next we lived and loved. For fun, we would walk along the water at the beach, then dinner at our favorite Mexican restaurant. We went dancing almost every Friday night. Joe loved jazz and we would dance all night. Sometimes when we were tired, our Friday night date would be take-out and a movie. We would curl up with each other and Riley on the couch, those nights were magic for us. Our private, sensual life continued to flourish. Joe could take my breath away with a look.

Between work, family parties, and holidays, our time together flew. We were in sync with each other. Our lives took on a rhythm much like a dance. We flowed from one moment to the next effortlessly. Staying in the moment was easy; Joe was my point of focus and delight.

Christmas and New Years were especially important to us, we had our first date Christmas Eve and New Year's Eve was our second date. The New Year always held the promise of hope and a bright future for us. When Joe and I declared our love for each other on our Wedding day, he promised me he would live and love me until he was one hundred years old. I was holding him to that promise. Each New Year, he would renew that promise.

Then without warning, our lives slowly began to change.

It was closing day on our new home. Our dream had finally come true. We were so excited, our own home, no more renting. We arrived at the tittle company eager to begin our life in our own home. Joe seemed confused when faced with all the documents, I had to show him where to sign each page and there were many! Another niggling of fear began to creep into the back of my mind. I chalked this feeling up to both of us being nervous and excited.

The first project was to paint the interior of our house. Before we hung the first picture, I asked Joe for a permanent black marker.

He said, "Why do you want a black marker?"

"I have lived in rentals most of my life, I always promised myself that if I ever had the privilege of owning my own home, I would write on the walls in permanent black ink."

With that said, he handed me the marker, and I wrote. "This is my house and I can write on the walls if I want to!" We both signed and dated our private message. Then we hung a picture of his mother over those precious words, she kept our secret for us.

The carpet was the original, about thirty years old! We proceeded to install new carpet and then clean up the yard, it was piled high with broken glass, wood and old plumbing supplies. We spent every waking moment, when we were not working, on our house. We had so much fun! We dug up all thirty of our roses from the rental and transplanted them in our new backyard.

After a few months, we bought chair rails and big four-inch baseboards to put in our home. When Joe went to the garage to start the project, he pulled out his miter saw and could not figure out how to unlock it. I had watched him do this simple task a thousand times, so I did it for him. He was confused and embarrassed that he could not do it for himself.

I became very quiet and my heart beat wildly in my chest, what was this? How could he not be able to use his beloved saw, which he had used for years? Something in the back of my mind began to make my skin crawl, but I pushed that feeling down deep into my subconscious.

I had never actually used his saw, even though he had shown me many times. I had no one to call for help, everyone in my family was busy and to tell the truth, I do not think I really wanted to tell them why I needed help. I dug deep trying to remember all that Joe had told me about his saw and how not to cut off my fingers.

I measured the walls carefully, went back to the garage, set the saw, said a prayer and made my first cut. I took the baseboard into the house to see if it fit. The baseboard fit perfectly! I was so shocked I could hardly contain myself. With Joe holding the baseboards in place, I used the nail gun and the portable compressor to nail them to the wall. By nightfall all, the baseboards were securely in place.

"Well done!" Joe said with pride. I beamed with humility, "How did I do that?"

Joe took my face in his hands and said, "You are so beautiful, I love you".

"It's so nice to be married to an old blind man!" I would say, and then we would hold each other and laugh.

However, this time it was tinged with a slow budding fear, which I couldn't ignore.

Joe and I were going to take a week of vacation to continue to work on our house. I worked all day to prepare the office for my vacation and as I said good-bye to my boss, he motioned me into his office.

I sat down, to update him on my day's preparations.

"Wanda, things have slowed down here and I can no longer afford to keep you."

Time stopped and my ears began to buzz white noise. My mouth went dry and I could barely speak, I said, "What! You're letting me go. I've been here for three years, why?"

"Yes, I'm sorry; I can't afford you any longer."

My boss got up from behind his desk and came to sit down next to me, I had gone white and felt faint, and he could see that.

"Are you ok, Wanda, I'm really sorry!"

"I just bought a house; you know that, I won't be able to pay my mortgage without this job! I asked you before I bought my house if my job with you was secure and you said, yes!"

He looked me square in the face, then lowered his eyes and said in a very quiet voice, "I know, here is your severance pay, I've added a few extra weeks. Have anyone call, I'll give you a good reference, you've done a great job here. I can't do anything about this, I'm sorry."

I turned on my heels and stomped out of his office. As I neared my car, I realized he hadn't asked me for my keys.

I marched back into his office, threw the keys across his desk, and said, "Hey, the next time you fire someone, be sure to get the office keys!"

Then I slowly walked out to my car, I could not feel my feet.

I cried all the way to Jim and Cheryl's; I was meeting Joe for dinner there to celebrate our vacation. I walked into their house and blurted out my bad news.

It stopped everyone in their tracks, no one spoke for a moment, then Joe rushed up to me, took me in his arms and said, "Don't worry, my love, we'll be all right. You are smart, you'll find another job, and then, he kissed me long and slow.

Jim and Cheryl gave me hugs, Cheryl offered me food, Jim offered me a drink; the rest of the evening was spent laughing as Jim recounted all the bad jobs he had had. He would do anything to make me feel better; boy, I loved that man.

After many sleepless nights and many tears, I found a new job in a large office. I was so relieved that I would be able to pay our mortgage that I was week with relief. I knew nothing about the work I was about to do, but was eager to learn. This was a stressful job and all consuming. I enjoyed meeting all my new clients and employees but worried that I had bitten off more than I could chew.

I was side tracked by having to find a new job so for a while, I stopped worrying about Joe's increasing memory problems. He seemed normal and I relaxed into our new routine. Evenings were peaceful, I was happy to ignore the outside world at night.

Joe put in for a transfer to the new hardware store that was opening near our home; it would mean that he would not have to commute. His company graciously granted Joe a transfer. He started out great, although Joe sometimes seemed a little confused when he would talk about his new store.

Joe would get lost, it was bigger, and it was a new environment. I was not concerned as they were still under construction and everything was chaotic, who would not get confused. Joe asked me one day to write his social security number on a piece of paper to keep in his wallet, he used that number to punch in on their time clock. That surprised me a little, but again I chalked it up to a new environment and a lot of stress.

He said, "Sometimes I am in such a hurry to punch in and the time clock doesn't always work right and I do not want to make others wait while I remember my number."

I said, "Of course." That seemed logical to me, but there was a slow tingling feeling in the back of my mind.

eleven

The Blessing

They come in many shapes and sizes.

They come in many colors.

Babies

God entrusts them to our care for just a little while.

Sometimes we forget that we can't keep them.

We raise them, love them and guide them.

Then, we must let them go.

While they become a reflection of us, they become

a reflection of themselves in God.

After we have let them go, we get to watch whom we have raised.

We get to see our love pour out of them, into their own lives.

If we are lucky, they come back to us as friends

to shine on forever in our lives.

As we grow old, these friends raise us, guide us and love us.

Then, they must let us go.

We then become a reflection of their love to shine down upon them forever.

Wanda

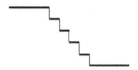

MARCH 2005

*I*t was early March, when, Abby showed up at my house with what I can only describe as a terrified look on her face. I was still reeling from Joe losing his job and all the tests to determine if he in fact, had Alzheimer's. My life had been a whirlwind of doctor's appointments and stress.

"Hi Abby, how are you, are you ok?"

She grabbed me in a big hug and began to cry.

"Mom, I can't believe this, you won't believe this; I am pregnant!"

"What!"

"Mom, how did this happen?" I began to laugh!

"Abby you are thirty years old, if you have to ask me that, then I know how you got pregnant!"

She laughed at me as she fell through the door and into my arms.

I held her and my heart swelled with pride, I was going to be a grandmother again. I was going to watch a baby grow as I watched my husband unravel. I sent a silent prayer to god. "Please, let me be able to handle all of this!"

"Come on Abby, this is unbelievably great news." I was thrilled!

She was so scared, she never even thought about having a baby, Abby had met Brady a longtime friend of the family and had quickly fallen head over heels in love with him.

"It's too soon, I am not ready yet!" she cried.

"Well, you and Brady better get ready this baby is coming and what a blessing for all of us!"

She laughed, and said, "Its ok then, that I have a baby?"

"Yes, there is always room in our hearts to love another baby!"

We sat and talked for a long time, reminiscing about her and Amy and our births, it was a wonderful mother/daughter bonding moment. I assured her that she and Brady would be wonderful parents.

As Abby left she said," "I am really going to need you, mom."

I hugged her and said, "Don't worry, Abby I'll be with you every step of the way."

With that, she danced off to her car, happy now to think about the prospect of motherhood. I believe she went shopping that afternoon, which always made Abby feel better!

After Abby left, I sat down and stared out the window. Another nice day, and how different it had become, I was going to be a grandmother again. I was so worried about Joe and now I had to think about Abby, how was I going to do this? How could I juggle happiness and sadness at the same time? You know what people say, "God never gives you more than you can handle." Really, really! Part of me wanted to laugh with delight, and part of me wanted to weep!

The whole family was ecstatic about the news of a new baby; it had been almost 10 years since Bailey was born. We were overdue for a new life in our family. Miracles were popping up all over the place. With that, I finally fell asleep.

JULY 2005

I woke up with a headache as I realized that I did not sleep much last night. Saying goodbye to Joe's children had been so emotional and exhausting. Lying awake most of the night reliving our past had not helped much either. Today I was back in the present and very tired.

I was still basking in the joy of being with Matt and Raechael. I needed to clean the house and meet Amy and Abby at the maternity store. Abby was growing out of all her clothes. I took Joe over to Jim's, so he did not have to spend the day alone.

It was so much fun to be with my daughters. We walked all over the mall, Abby with her hands resting on her swelling belly, complaining about how fat she looked and Amy looking for cute new clothes for her new niece! This was the best part of motherhood. I laughed at their antics all day. We had so many bags by the end of our little excursion; I could barely get them in our car!

I got a call from Abby on Bailey's tenth birthday; she was in labor. What are the odds that twin girls give birth exactly ten years apart? Abby was very nervous, but excited to be giving birth. Brady was pacing, but appeared surprisingly calm! Joe and I raced to the rescue!

Amy was already there when we arrived and was instructing Abby to stay calm! Bailey was anxious to share her birthday with her new little cousin. Bailey had grown into such an intelligent young girl. She was emotionally way beyond her years with beautiful with deep green eyes, ringed with thick long black lashes. Her face covered with creamy white skin sported a square jaw, Joe's jaw.

This was going to be a crazy, but exciting day. Joe did not really understand what was going on as we told him he was going to be a grandfather, but he grinned from ear to ear.

It took Abby two days to deliver Harlyn; she was beautiful and big 9 lbs. Abby had a very hard delivery, which took its toll on all of us. I felt every labor pain and pushed every push with her. Harlyn swallowed mucosa and was admitted to the Neo Natal unit of the hospital. Brady never left the side of his baby girl.

"Mom, will she be alright, will my baby girl live?" Abby cried.

"Yes, Abby, this happens to babies, sometimes, she will be all right. We'll be with her every day; God won't let anything happen to your baby!"

I silently prayed, "God please, please wrap your Angels wings around Harlyn, give her back to her mother! I can't watch my daughter go through this agony, please God help us!" After seven grueling days, Harlyn was home with her parents.

As this was Abby and Brady's first baby, Harlyn was with me a lot. Joe loved his new baby; he would feed her and rock her for hours. I never left him alone with Harlyn, but would sit and watch Joe love her. He would kiss and nuzzle her neck and speak softly to her. His words did not always make sense but Harlyn did not mind.

My new little granddaughter was perfect in every way. Her parents were loving, caring and filled with the joys a new baby brings to your life. I watched my little baby grow and I watched Joe fall down those proverbial stairs. With each breath, I was enthralled and shocked at the same time. Sometimes, I would hold Harlyn and at the same time hold Joe's hand as he struggled to make sense of his once normal life.

As Joe once told me," Watch the signs, Wanda, watch the signs." To me, that meant everything happens for a reason, it would not be until much later that I would understand his words.

twelve

"Sometimes, I felt like I was in the middle of a lake,
trying to swim to the shore with an anchor tied around my
ankle. Then I would pray, "Please get me safely to the shore."
I would find myself buoyed up and floating peacefully."

Wanda

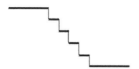

AUGUST 2005 – MAY 2009

I would go to work in the morning and Joe would stay home by himself, he would walk Riley and work in his garden. I would make him lunch and leave it in the refrigerator. I gave him strict instructions not to go anywhere other than the neighborhood, and he agreed. I gave him a cell phone and I called him every two hours to check on him. Joe always answered the phone; he was happy and cheerful so I did not need to worry.

I called every agency I could think of to see what kind of help I could get for Joe. That turned out to be a nightmare. I made too much money for any financial aid, most agencies could not help, however they were very sympathetic to my situation. I was fifty-two and still needed to work. Joe was fifty-eight and would need twenty-four hour care soon. I made a good living, but I could not afford to hire someone to come into our home to take care of him. Putting him in a convalescent hospital was out of the question.

The only thing I was able to do was adult daycare. The problem with that was they opened at 9am. I left my house at 6:45am and they closed at 2pm. I worked until 5pm and had a forty-five minute commute. I was the office manager at my office and could not be away from my job to be sick, let alone in and out for Joe.

During my quest to find help, one woman on the phone asked me where Joe was now. I told her that he was still able to be home alone.

She said in a stern voice, "Do you realize that if he gets hurt at home you could be found guilty of negligence?"

I gasped, "What?"

"Yes", she said, "Because you know he has Alzheimer's, it is like leaving a young child home alone, you could be in big trouble!"

I thanked her profusely and left work early, my legs felt rubbery as I jumped in my car pulled away from the curb and raced home.

I bolted through the door, yelling Joe's name, there was no answer, and I quickly raced through each room of our very small house, no Joe. I opened the sliding door out to our patio and I heard him whistling in his rose garden, he was all right; I had not killed him with my ignorance.

I had to get a grip and some help! After he gave me a big hug, he was always so happy to see me; I sat down with the phone book to look for adult day care.

The only one that made any sense was near my work; however, what was I going to do with him before 9am and after 2pm? My office was great, my boss said I could bring Joe to work and then bring him back after 2pm. Problem solved.

I took Joe to the kitchen to watch movies while I worked. This arrangement was so incredibly kind of my office; however, this drove me crazy. I was constantly checking on him. Joe would get tired of the small confines of the kitchen. I finally gave him a job; he loved odd jobs. I would let him pick up fallen leaves in the parking lot. That worked for a while but I was constantly running to the lobby to check on him, I was scared he would wander into the street.

I became depressed, and frantic, I really did not know what to do with him. My children, and Jim and Cheryl worked so; they could not help me. I knew my job was suffering, however no one dared say so, the whole office felt so sorry for me. Joe was very sweet and happy, everyone would spoil him; our staff would bring him treats, which he loved since his main hobby had always been eating.

Joe had always gotten up early to experience first light, so starting the day early was easy for him. The hard part was with me, I had two people to get ready in the morning. We would sing and laugh all the way to work. He was very happy to be with me at work in the morning. Joe loved coffee so he was happy for another cup and a doughnut.

However going to day care was another issue. Joe did not like day care. I had to pry him out of the car every morning. I would walk in with him, show him around, and tell him to help the people. Joe loved helping and that would appease him somewhat. I would kiss him and promise I would be back very soon.

In order to get him comfortable I would have to sit him with another person who he could talk to, he had become very chatty lately. Joe would start a conversation with anyone who would stand still and listen. Some days Joe would see me leave and he would follow me to the front door and cry as I got in the car. This was horrible and I would cry all the way back to work. My day care solution was not working. I was frantic for a solution. I do not think I have ever felt so alone and helpless. Praying constantly I asked, "Please God, help me help Joe."

thirteen

"Surprises come in the ordinary moments of our lives. That is where the blessings are, that is where love resides. That is where God lives."

Wanda

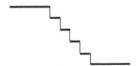

*T*he phone rang early on a Saturday morning. "Hi Wanda, this is Raechael."

"Hi, how are you?" I was always so excited to hear from her. We had become fast friends. Raechael was always so honest and upbeat, she was fun to talk with.

"Matt and I are great, I have exciting news!" she rushed forward. "Matt and I are having a baby!"

Raechael and Matt had been married the year before and were ready to include a baby into their lives. I was so excited, you would have thought this was going to be my own biological grandbaby, the lines were blurry when it came to Joe's kids, I felt like they were mine!

"Oh Raechael, I'm so happy for you and Matt, it's time for some good news. Joe's going to be so excited!"

I put Joe on the phone, Raechael got Matt and father and son talked for a long time.

I was not sure Joe understood about the baby.

"Joey, do you understand that Matt and Raechael are going to have a baby, he'll be your first grandchild?"

"Yes!" he said and smiled like a Cheshire cat!

Elijah Joseph Proost was born in December.

When Raechael called to tell us about the birth, she asked to talk to Joe.

"Hi Joe, this is Raechael, our baby was born today, it's a boy. Matt and I are naming him Elijah Joseph Proost, after you. Do you understand?"

Joe grinned and nodded into the phone. We all started crying, another miracle. It was so poignant of Matt and Raechael to give Elijah Joe's name.

Our granddaughters, Bailey and Harlyn were growing so fast. Bailey, in grammar school was a smart, quick witted, beautiful young girl. She reminded me so much of her mother and her aunt Abby. Bailey was a perfect blending of my two daughters. Harlyn was walking and now talking, she was a beautiful little cherub. She had a cute round face with creamy white skin and big brown eyes. Her first words came out as sentences and she spoke like a child much older than her years. Bailey and Harlyn were inseparable; they were more like sisters than cousins.

Joe was doing just the opposite, and his speech was becoming harder to understand. His words did not always make sense. He loved the girls and would sit and talk with them for hours; they seemed to understand each other perfectly. Joe love cartoons and the three of them would sit and snuggle; I loved hearing their squeals of laughter. Bailey too old for cartoons would sit patiently with Joe always attentive, she watched out for him.

Joe was losing himself fast! I talked to Jim and Cheryl and we decided to go on a two-week vacation together. We knew it would be Joe's last vacation. It was important to Cheryl and me that Jim and Joe spend as much time together as possible. I had been so stressed out that I needed a break, so what better way to rest than a vacation. Jim and Cheryl had just bought a fifth wheel and a new truck. We were off to the Delta for a camping vacation!

Joe and I got up early Saturday morning. I remember thinking how light hearted and normal I felt as I loaded our suitcases and camping gear into our car. It had been such a long time since I felt like that. Spending time with Jim and Cheryl made me feel safe. I was genuinely excited. We loaded up the fifth wheel with food, fishing gear, and enough camping equipment to supply many families. As usual, we were very prepared!

Jim was driving, I was riding shotgun as I get car sick, and Cheryl and Joe were in the back seat. It only took Joe and Cheryl a few minutes to fall asleep, they looked so cute in the back seat huddled together sharing the same pillow. Meanwhile I was up front watching Jim drive. I am not a very good back seat driver, more than once I had to swallow the urge to tell Jim to be careful or slow down! Concentrating on Jim's driving kept me in the moment that day.

We were about half way to the Delta when Jim came very close to an accident. Driving way to fast with a 32-foot fifth wheel attached to his pick-up he had to slam on the breaks to avoid hitting the truck in front of us. I did not say a word, I instead just stopped breathing, and he did too!

After about five minutes, he turned to look at me and said, "Well, that went well, don't you think?"

I nervously laughed and said as I shook my head at him, "Oh my God, Jim!"

We both laughed. It is a good thing I loved that man, when we finally got to our campsite I was grateful to still be alive!

The four of us settled in and began two weeks of fun, fishing, eating way to much food and lots of reminiscing. Jim and Joe went fishing most every day. The only thing that Jim caught was a fishing pole and reel. He was excited, as it was a very expensive reel. Joe caught a three-inch baby fish that we promptly sent back into the Delta. We had neighbors bringing us their fresh caught fish; it became a joke in the campground, as they felt sorry for us. Cheryl and I were the only wives that could not cook our own fresh caught fish. Sometimes, Jim would buy fish at the local supermarket and pretend he caught it, no one believed him.

We met many wonderful campers and generally had a great time. Joe was so relaxed that he seemed better. I will always cherish those two weeks, for Jim and Joe the time spent together was priceless.

When the time came to go home, Jim, Cheryl and I were sad. Somehow, we had managed to stay in the moment during our vacation. However, now we knew we would never go on another trip together; the time ahead seemed gloomy. Reality was right around the corner and with no hope in sight, my heart felt heavy. I know Jim and Cheryl felt the same way, only Joe could be heard laughing, he had no idea what the future held.

Joe was beginning to step down those stairs again; he could not always find the towel closet and sometimes he would stand by the front door ready to go out without pants. Dressing Joe was becoming a big challenge and sometimes very funny. One morning he walked into the kitchen with his shirt on his head. We both laughed and I helped him fix it. Small things really, but they were very disconcerting.

Stay in the moment, Wanda, I would say to myself. To accomplish this I would engage Joe in a hug to ground me.

fourteen

"Sometimes, we are forced to make tough decisions, that later turn out to be blessings in disguise. Listen to your heart that is God talking to you."

Wanda

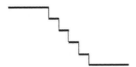

bout a week after we got back from our vacation, my boss asked me not to bring Joe back to work. He was pulling down his pants to tuck in his shirt and one of our office staff saw him and thought he was going to expose himself to her. I was embarrassed and upset, but I understood. This had not been the best situation for my office and while I really appreciated all of their help, it was time for me to make other arrangements.

That night I made a decision that I knew was coming, I would have to quit my job to take care of Joe. I was a little torn; I had worked very hard all my life and had a stellar resume. Now, I would be unemployed with a very sick husband. However, I did not want to miss the days we had left, they were precious. In the end, my decision was easy. Now, all I had to do was find a job where I could take Joe with me. You cannot imagine how upset my office was when I went to work the next day and quit.

My boss kept saying that I could not quit. I reminded him that I had no choice; I had no one to take care of Joe. I gave them two weeks' notice; it was the longest two weeks of my life. You cannot imagine how happy Joe was when I told him I had quit my job to stay home with him. I do not really know how much he understood, but I know he understood no more daycare. He actually said, "Yeah!" From that day on, he rarely left my side.

I had no job, but a very happy, very sick husband. I was unbelievably scared, yet strangely peaceful. I was doing what I had to do. I was helping my White Knight down the stairs of life; I was becoming his White Knight.

Miracles began to happen, I tried selling newspapers, and I started an on line business. I made some money but not enough to survive long term. The miracle was how far my meager earnings began to stretch. Mostly, I loved being with Joe every day. I was unbelievably busy as I worked and took care of the house all by myself. Joe was now just watching me and touching me when he could. I was happy in a terrified sort of way. I was in the moment most of the time now; I did not have time to look into the future.

fifteen

*"Never underestimate the power of family. We are given these
wonderful, if sometimes challenging people, to enrich and stabilize us.
Love comes in many forms; our responsibility is to see our families as
support from above. Love unconditionally and see the humor in all things."*

Wanda

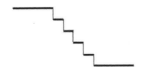

We began to spend Saturdays and most Sundays with Jim and Cheryl. They were such a huge source of love and support, no two people knew us better. When Joe was with them, they treated him like a normal man. Jim and Joe would always have a project of some kind in the garage or the yard, Jim was so patient with his brother. Cheryl and I would spend the day shopping and cooking elaborate dinners. Cheryl was an excellent cook and both Jim and Joe loved to eat, being with them was always a party. It made me feel normal and safe somehow. When I was with Jim, I always felt like everything would be ok, even though it was fleeting.

Jim and Cheryl had a small dinner party one night and invited Curtis and Eddie along with Joe and me. Their house was warm and inviting, and everyone was in high spirits. Joe reacting to the happy environment was relaxed and very chatty. Cheryl was busy in the kitchen, making her famous paella. Curtis and Eddie had known Jim and Cheryl for twenty-five years and were dear friends. Everyone was mingling and sharing stories about their families.

Jim invited Curtis out to the garage to see his latest purchase; I tagged along. Joe was always in the kitchen waiting for food, he stayed close to Cheryl. Eddie was chatting about her day, so I felt safe in escaping with the men. I could use a five-minute break.

Jim's garage, filled with tools, saws and his dogs, was a comforting place to hide out. Over in the corner, next to their freezer stood his latest purchase and his pride and joy, a five-foot high shiny black safe.

Jim proudly told Curtis, "I haven't been feeling very strong lately and I was worried that if we had an intruder, I couldn't protect Cheryl. So, I bought a 357 magnum and a riffle."

Curtis now sat forward and said, "Wow! Jim, you bought new guns?"

"Yes, I hope I'll never need them, but if I do I'll be ready!"

I already knew about the guns and was a little nervous that Jim had so much firepower in his possession. Jim stepped up to the safe, with his back to us began to spin the dial, and began to use the combination. Two turns to the right, two turns to the left. Jim looked over his shoulder at me, as if he thought I might steal his combination!

Again, he set himself in front of the dial, three turns to the right, two turns to the left, nothing. He looked over at me and I looked down. He started over and I began to laugh. It was obvious to Curtis and me that he had forgotten the combination. Curtis' body was shaking with suppressed laughter. Jim looked back at me for the third time and I could no longer contain myself!

"Having trouble, Jim?" I asked swallowing a barely concealed laugh.

Jim stepped away from the safe, now Curtis and I were laughing aloud. Jim started laughing at himself.

"Hey, Jim where is the ammunition?" I asked.

"Well, under the bed."

"So, if you have an intruder, you have to grab the bullets from under the bed, run down the hallway and out to the garage. Open the safe with the combination, that you can't remember, load your handgun, then run back in the house and tell the intruder, Stop! I have a gun?" I asked giggling.

Jim thought for a moment and said, "Yes!"

That was all it took for all of us to laugh until we could not breathe.

When Cheryl called us into dinner, we were exhausted! The rest of the night, we spent laughing at my crazy, crazy brother-in-law. Curtis did not get to see Jim's guns that night.

That Christmas was hard for me; Joe did not seem to understand what was going on. He did not participate in the decorating; going with me to buy presents was confusing to him. Christmas Eve and Christmas Day he spent sitting in a corner, he did not interact with anyone. My heart broke as I stayed next to him as much as my family would allow.

My family would sneak sorrowful glances in my direction when they thought I was not looking. I knew they felt sorry for me and I think that was the worst. I did not feel sorry for myself, rather a love so fierce for Joe that I sometimes thought my heart would burst. It was impossible to put into words the feelings I was experiencing. I so wanted Joe to be able to enjoy those simple pleasures that were once such a natural part of his life, the very ones my family took so easily for granted. Our days were numbered and I knew it. Staying in the moment was impossible for me that Christmas.

sixteen

"Words of wisdom, always listen to your mother!
Sometimes your children give you gifts of wisdom, listen to them.
God speaks to you through the people you love the most."

Wanda

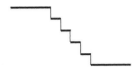

*I*t was clear to me that I needed a better paying job. Once again, I was faced with the dilemma of earning a living with Joe by my side.

My mom said to me one day," You were an operations manager for a janitorial company, why don't you clean houses?"

"Oh, God, housework?" I groaned, wasn't I already doing the housework of two people?

"You're probably right, mom, but how will I get clients? I would have to get a business license, advertise, and buy equipment. I don't know if I have the energy, I'm so tired. I'll sleep on it."

I slept on it and realized that I had no choice. Now, so many hurdles, start a business, get a business license, buy insurance, find clients, and all while Joe followed me around like a puppy. I was already so tired the future seemed insurmountable.

I did what I have always done when faced with a problem, put one foot in front of the other, and look up. Two weeks later, my Cleaning Company was born. I was licensed, bonded, and insured. My company became a family affair, mom gave me the idea, Amy chose the name and Abby helped me with advertising.

I bought equipment, cleaning supplies, business cards, and I immediately starting getting clients. Within a month, my schedule was full. I usually only worked in the mornings, Joe needed to be home in the afternoons and eight hours of cleaning was too much for me.

Joe went with me every day; in the beginning he vacuumed, he loved that. Sometimes I worried he was going to vacuum the pile right off the carpets, he would vacuum for hours. He felt important and it really did help me. The rest of the time, he would follow me around and watch me clean. It was stressful for me because he did not have good spacial skills. I was always worried that he would break something, but low and behold, I was the only one breaking things! All my clients loved Joe; they would spoil him with cookies and baked goods, sometimes he could be seen sleeping in their rocking chairs.

Joe was beginning to fall from his plateau again. He would stabilize for a few months then there would be a sharp drop in cognitive skills and he would stabilize again at the lower level. Helping Joe step down the stairs of life was a pattern that would stay with us until the end. I could almost tell when he was going to drop down the stairs. It was grueling for me.

I began to notice that taking a shower had become too much for him, sometimes he would get out of the shower with soapy hair. I solved that problem by taking a shower with him every day. I had been dressing him for a quite a while. Joe continued to try to dress himself but pants, shoes, and socks were hard.

Picking up after Riley had become a challenge as he refused to wear gloves. Sometimes, he would wear them and then throw them away with the dog poop. I cannot tell you the number of times I had to wash his hands in alcohol. He would just look at me and sigh, as though I was a pain in his behind! He loved Riley, and got so much pleasure from taking care of him, that I would just laugh and buy more alcohol and gloves.

Joe and I both loved movies, I rented them all the time, when the credits came on at the end of the movie and the music began to play he would grab my hand and pull me close and dance around the living room, he still was quite romantic. That also became a problem.

The last time we made love it was more like a rape to me. Joe had forgotten how to play nice and the abruptness of it was too much for me to handle emotionally. I decided we were done with the physical side to our marriage. I wanted to remember the fabulous times, not this time. It was not Joe's fault, just another causality of this horrendous disease.

I took that sensual part of me and locked it away for safekeeping. I began to wear flannel to bed and I would wait until he fell asleep to crawl in next to him. I appeased his appetite by our showers in the mornings; Joe could hardly wait for his morning showers. His temperament stayed even and peaceful and, easy to bathe, thank God!

New Year's Eve was becoming bittersweet for me. While the whole world was looking forward to a better future, I knew my next year was going to get worse. I was scared of the unknown. I knew millions of people in the world felt scared, but for me this was a new experience. No matter what life had dealt me, I could always see a way to a more positive future. Now, however, I was a prisoner of Alzheimer's. I sometimes felt like I had the disease, it so colored my every move. Sometimes, I could not see the difference between Joe and me.

"Stay in the moment Wanda, stay in the moment!" I would say to myself as I headed for the kitchen to prepare a feast, including cake for New Year's Eve. In order to enjoy the night, I cooked a lavish meal, snuggled, and watched a comedy with Joe. I did not look ahead to tomorrow let alone the coming year. I felt every minute and concentrated on my sensory perceptions. Touching Joe helped me feel him emotionally somehow, breathing in his essence slowed my pulse and calmed me.

When the front door of my house shut at night and I put on the flip lock, so Joe could not escape. I would look around the house and realize that no matter how much my family wanted to help me in the end it was just Joe and me. It was in those times that I would pray for peace and guidance.

"Dear God, please wrap your Angels wings around us, please send the white light of the Holy Spirit to fill my heart with love and patience, please help me, help, Joe."

I sometimes prayed aloud. Joe would come up to me, put his head on my shoulder and hold me. Then, I would cry.

seventeen

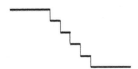

$\mathcal{J}$im and Joe were taking a large pick-up load of junk to the dump, Jim collected everything and getting him to go to the dump was an act of congress! They loaded a couch on top of the heap.

"Jim, are you going to tie down that couch?" I asked innocently.

"No, it will be fine. It is sitting there securely and will not go anywhere!"

He said shaking his head at me. "You worry too much!"

Joe was busy adding little bits and pieces to the load, he loved going to the dump.

Cheryl sighed, "Yeah, Jim knows everything, of course they should tie down the couch, you know, Wanda he will not listen to you!"

Cheryl and I walked back in the house to cook shaking our heads at our crazy husbands!

When the boys got home, Jim said, "When we got to the dump, the couch was gone, we retraced our path but couldn't find it!"

Joe said, "Yep, it was gone."

Cheryl and I did not want to say I told you so, but we did! We all just laughed; someone probably thought it was Christmas. Jim and Joe were shocked that it fell off the truck. Things like that happened all the time; they never listened to us.

As Cheryl walked back into the kitchen she said, "You know, that's how dumb Jim is, if was me, I never would have admitted that to him."

Joe was having trouble recognizing when he had to use the bathroom, so he would not make it. I was scrubbing up after him, just like a little puppy. I finally had to make the decision, that now he needed diapers. It was another downturn for us, another step down the stairs. This was another sign to me that our time was growing short.

I first tried adult diapers, but I could not get them to stay on, so I switched to pull on diapers and they worked perfectly. Joe thought they were jockeys. Problem solved.

Matt and Raechael brought Elijah for his first visit with his grandpa. I started marking days off on the calendar so Joe could see he was coming. When I would talk about his grandson, Joe would get excited, then, he would forget him. I prayed that Joe would be receptive to his new baby and would make Matt and Raechael feel welcome. Joe surpassed all my expectations as they knocked on our door that beautiful spring day.

Raechael stood there holding Elijah and said, "Hi, Joe, this is your grandson Elijah!"

Joe reached for his little five-month-old baby, took him lovingly in his arms and kissed him on the head. Joe knew who he was and held him until Elijah cried out for food. Matt was so proud, that he could not stop grinning.

Jim and Cheryl, Amy, Andon and Bailey, Abby, Brady and Harlyn came over for dinner. We all had so much fun, our family dinners were always lively, and we laughed until our cheeks hurt.

Now, we had two babies and a pre-teen in our normally quiet home. It was a flurry of dirty diapers and bottles. Bailey was such a big help feeding and playing with her little cousins. That night for just a few hours, my life seemed normal. It was the first time

I had all three of my grandchildren under one roof, I was so proud. I was in the moment the whole time.

Matt and Raechael spent a week with us; loving Joe and watching Joe love Elijah. Joe was never far from his little baby. Towards the end of the week, I could see Jim and Joe both slowing down. The week filled with dinners and sight-seeing and had taken its toll on the two brothers.

The good-byes were filled with last minute pictures and tears. We were not sure when we would see Matt and Raechael again, I was so sad to see them leave.

I had to struggle to stay in the moment that night. I started to feel depressed as I realized that our situation was becoming dire, and I felt very alone. We snuggled on the couch to watch a movie sharing a bag of popcorn. Joe fell asleep; I spent the rest of the evening memorizing his face. I stroked his sleeping hand and breathed in the essence of him. I relaxed into the moment with my White Knight.

eighteen

"Life can surprise you, it is imperative to stay flexible and feel each moment."

Wanda

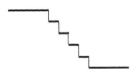

*J*im called one night and asked. "Hey, let's go out to dinner."

"Tonight, really?" "Yes, that would be great! I was just standing in front of the refrigerator, not knowing what to cook!"

It had been a long time since we had all gone out together; I was in the mood for a little fun. I could use a thick, juicy steak and a glass of wine. I was tired and hungry.

"Meet you at our favorite restaurant in half an hour." He said.

"Thank you, Jim, great idea!" See you there!"

The restaurant is a pub like bar with a cozy, old world feel. The food was amazing and populated by the locals.

Jim and Cheryl were already sitting in a booth when we arrived, hugs and kisses were exchanged and we sat down. I noticed how loud and busy it was, of course, it was a Friday night. I could feel Joe's body tense as we scooted in the booth.

Our server came to get our drink order, wine for me, and diet coke for Joe. I was starving so I started looking at the menu. Joe could not understand what food was by asking, so I would order two dinners that I thought he would like. I would let Joe choose what he wanted to eat when the meals were served. This worked out good for us; he was always excited to pick his dinner.

Joe chose the chicken and I got the steak. I helped him with his napkin and watched as he struggled to choose what silverware to use.

"Here, Joey, let me help you." I picked up his knife and fork for him.

He smiled at me as I put them in the wrong hands; he was left-handed.

As we ate, Joe became increasingly upset. At first, we all kept talking, trying to pretend that everything was ok. Joe finally, took his plate, shoved it at Jim, and tried to push me out of the booth. "Go, go!" he shouted.

He had had enough and wanted to go home.

Joe caught me off guard; he had never acted like this before. I put my arms around him and in a soft voice said, "Its ok, Joey, we're ok. Let's finish dinner and we'll go home."

I kept stroking his face and whispering in his ear that he was all right, finally he calmed down. We quickly finished dinner and left.

It was still early and Joe was very happy to be back in the car, so we went to Jim and Cheryl's for desert. We spent the rest of the evening in laughter as Jim reminisced about "the old days", while Joe joined in the laughter. I do not think Joe always understood everything Jim said but he always laughed when Jim did.

As we left, Jim said. "I guess no more dinners out."

Sadly, I agreed. When in an unfamiliar environment, with Alzheimer's, the patient does not know what is happening next and the hubbub of a crowded restaurant creates too much stress.

Shopping also became a challenge. We were in a grocery store standing in line at 5pm one evening. Joe got so upset that he started pushing our cart into the woman's cart in front of us.

"Move, move!" Joe shouted. The woman looked at us as if we were crazy. I tried to back up, but; there were five carts behind us. We were stuck.

The checker was about to call security, when I said in a quiet voice, "I am so sorry, my husband has Alzheimer's. I had to hold onto Joe to calm him down. Joe looked so normal that it seemed to her that we were simply impatient. The woman huffed and puffed until she left, giving me a dirty look as she stomped away. I was very embarrassed and wanted to cry. The checker looked at me with pity in his eyes. No more grocery stores, Joe had boxed me in, how was I to function and not take him with me.

I kept adjusting my life to accommodate Joe and after a while, I became an extension of him and could not find the person I used to be. Everything had changed so much and the scary thing was that I got used to it. I was falling into Alzheimer's, no day for me was normal, yet everything seemed normal. I was always in the moment now, one step down at a time. I began to forget Wanda. This moment-to-moment living was good for Joe, not always easy for me. When I needed to go shopping, I had to take Joe to Jim and Cheryl's, which gave me a little break. The spontaneity of just running to the store was over, now even the simplest shopping spree had to be preplanned.

There were times when I would forget that Joe was sick. One afternoon, I was taking a shower as I turned off the water; I realized I had forgotten a towel.

I yelled, "Joey will you please get me a towel?"

He said, "Ok!"

I waited patiently, minutes went by and no towel.

Again, I yelled, "Joey, will you please get me a towel?"

Again, he yelled back, "Ok!"

I was beginning to get cold, instead of going to get my own towel; I proceeded to give him directions to the linen closet. Finally, after I was almost completely dry I realized that he was never going to bring me a towel. I stood there laughing at myself! I had to get my own towel.

The one thing that helped me keep sane was my love for Joe. As long as I kept my eye on the ball and kept his routine simple and predictable life, with him was very easy. I was the one that sometimes complicated my life. Here is another funny story.

I was showering alone one morning and just as I turned off the shower and grabbed for a towel Joe popped his head into the bathroom and stood there opened mouthed.

I said, "What's wrong Joey?"

He said nothing. I kept drying off, he left and came right back and did another double take. This time, I realized as he stood there staring at me dripping wet that he had never seen a naked woman before.

He left and came back two more times before I actually got embarrassed and said, "Get out of here!"

Later, now dressed I laughed; it had not occurred to me that it was as if Joe was a young boy again! I had to be careful what he saw, Oh God, the challenges never ended.

That attitude worked in my favor at dinner, however. No matter what I put in front of him to eat, he looked at it as if it was his first meal. All those meals that should have been boring for him became feasts that he would try for the first time.

Every meal ended with, "That was the best food I've ever had!"

Dinner was easy until… one night I gave Joe a bowl of soup, a salad and a hot dog. In order to eat it he needed a fork, spoon and his fingers. We were sitting at our coffee table to eat and watch a movie. Joe stared at his plate and his fork and spoon. Picking up the spoon, he tried to put his hot dog on it, and then he tried to eat his soup with his fork. I gently tried to help him; he pulled away becoming very frustrated. I backed off and left him alone to figure dinner out for himself. As you can imagine, it was a disaster. Finally, he let me help him, after that, I made sure that whatever I was having for dinner needed only one utensil. Another step down the stairs.

That dinner was a reminder that small day-to-day events for me were overwhelming for Joe. A lesson I never forgot, I became very sensitive to what he perceived. These events were jarring for me and shook me to my core.

I asked him one day what it felt like to be Joe Proost, he thought for a minute, grinned and said, "I feel great, I feel clear, everything is so clear for me."

I think what Joe meant was that his mind was uncluttered. There was no "normal" chatter going on inside his mind. We are constantly thinking and reliving our pasts, and looking to the future, real or imagined. We spend a goodly amount of time worrying about things that almost never happen. With an Alzheimer's patient, they do not remember the past and cannot imagine the future. Actually, they only see the present, literally and because of that, their minds are clear.

These childlike victims are upset and scared if we as caregivers expect too much of them. I found if I stayed in the present with Joe everything rolled along calmly. I was the only one to upset him if I expected too much or moved to fast.

Since I am a triple A personality, it taught me a lesson and to this day I continue to stay in the present (most of the time). Joe taught me that I was wasting the present by either looking back or looking forward. Alzheimer's patients really have a lot to teach us, if we stop to listen.

As you, carefully guide your Alzheimer's patient down the stairs of life. You need to be in the moment so as not to trip on the stairs yourself. The most effective way for me was to anchor myself with him. I would look at the world through his eyes. Feeling each moment in front of me was the key. If you are feeling each moment, you are in it.

Remember how you saw the world through your young children's eyes. How everything was fresh and new. It is the same with an Alzheimer's patient; to them everything is fresh and new. They see the world as brand new in each moment; see the world with them and watch your experience change. Your frustration lessens, your impatience lessens you begin to see the miracle of a moment.

nineteen

I promise------

When you are sad, I will make you laugh.

When you have dark days, I will hold you close

until the sun comes out in your eyes.

When you laugh, I will laugh with you.

When you need loving, I will give my body and soul to you.

When you walk in the sand, I will match you step for step.

When you fall behind me, I will stop and wait for you.

When you need encouragement, I will gently nudge your tender spirit.

When you ask for forgiveness, I will forgive you.

When you need quiet, I will be still.

When you need me, I will always be there.

This I promise you.

Wanda

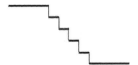

That night I went to bed and had an unbelievable dream:

The question that I had asked Joe was; "What does it feel like to be you?"

His answer surprised me, "Clear, I feel very clear, my mind is free, I have no worries. I feel better than I ever have in my whole life. "Come, come my darling, be with me!"

I had never met anyone that had no worries; I wanted to be him, to feel what he was feeling, to see what he saw, to know what he knew. This is where my journey began.

I was standing in our garden, surrounded by Joe's beautiful and fragrant roses, when no sooner had I thought about what it would be like to be him than I began to feel peculiar. There was a tingling in my arms and feet. My insides felt like they were collapsing, I was not in pain, but scared to death. What was going on? I looked at the ground as it rushed up to meet me, I thought I was fainting, but I did not lose consciousness. All of a sudden, the world seemed much bigger to me. The roses were now towering over my head like the skyscrapers, in New York. I seemed to be the same size, but my world became overwhelmingly huge. My clothes still fit, blue jeans, white sweat shirt and white tennis shoes, so what had happened?

All of a sudden, I felt sucked into a strange and scary place. I looked around and all I could see were blood vessels, bones and tendons. Where was I? Oh! I could feel Joe, but now from the inside! A creepy crawly sensation began to nibble at the outer corner of my psyche, had I somehow willed myself into Joe's body. This was not as scary as I had anticipated; it was actually comforting somehow.

The light that shown through his eyes was brighter on the inside. Warm and welcoming, it was almost liquid and it glowed with pure joy. It helped me "see" as I started in his feet; they were sturdy, well formed; his toes wiggled easily, which made me laugh. Now, I was laughing from the inside/out, this was such a warm easy laugh, which bubbled up from my toes and reverberated through my whole body. How had I gotten so small? I fit in his feet and toes!

As I made my way up inside his legs, I noticed I had to move from side to side dodging his strong, sinewy muscles. From here, I could feel his power, his strength, it was amazing, and it felt like I could hold onto his ropey muscles and swing from them, first one then another. I began to climb up towards his thighs. I was amazed at the energy I had. Over developed from years of squatting, his thighs seemed so dense that I did not think they would let me pass on my journey. Upon closer inspection, they were actually softer than I expected, filled with red blood cells which buoyed me towards my next surprise.

I came to the area of life, the unexpected pleasure of human kind, the place held dear by all men. The pure sensuality of the experience astounded me. I could not spend too much time here, as I became enthralled with the most spine tingling, erotic feelings seducing me with wave upon wave of emotion unparralled on my earthy plane. This place was warm, warmth that spread through me and buoyed my spirit; I was floating, I did not want to leave. I was used to being in this place on the outside but here I felt like blushing.

I did not have to go far to reach his stomach, I could see inside, do not ask me how. I began to laugh; there were cupcakes, chips, candy buoyed in a sea of diet Pepsi. I did not see one vegetable, no fruit, nothing that would have suggested a healthy diet, yet so far, his body was strong and robust. I needed to move on; I was becoming hungry just being near all those carbs. Eating had always been an event, a kind of erotic dance we would do in the kitchen when preparing a meal. This was all the junk food he sneaked when I was not looking. I had to smile; he could still surprise me.

I must be getting close, I could hear the faint ta tum, ta tum, the beating of his heart. As I got closer, his heart rhythm sped up as he anticipated my arrival. This was a very familiar sound. I had spent hours with my head nestled on his chest, now from the inside I could watch his heart beat for me. It was a glorious feeling. I wrapped my tiny arms around his dark red smooth heart and held on for dear life. Quite a difference from the inside out, but so very comforting. As long as his heart was beating, my heart could beat in time with his. I stayed resting on his heart for a long time, not anxious to continue my travels. The beating slowed down, he let out a sigh of peace, and he did not want me to move either. We were so comfortable with each other, so in tune. This is what it was like to be in synchronicity with another human being.

I left the comfort of his heart slowly not really wanting to go, but knowing my journey was far from over I began reluctantly inward. I knew I was close to his lungs as I could feel the rhythmic movement in and out of his breath. Joe's chest would expand then contract, powerful in its exchange. I could barely stay still. This was the breath of life, the exchange of oxygen and carbon dioxide. I always marveled that as human beings, we live on oxygen, and the plant world lived on our expelling carbon dioxide. A perfect marriage, Joe was happy and he started to whistle. The sound rushed all around me, my hair began to blow all about my face, and I started to whistle too, not even realizing I was keeping time with him.

As I moved up towards his eyes, I wondered what I would see. Before I got there, Joe ate another snickers bar, which almost killed me. It threatened to drag me back to his stomach. I had to press myself against the inside of his throat, the big, sticky glob just missing my head, ugh! Not, so pretty from this vantage point, I was becoming a little scared.

As soon as he stopped swallowing, I slowly slithered up into his eyes, no telling what he might eat next! Wow! What a view, this was breathtaking. Joe was standing in his rose garden admiring his roses. They were beautiful, each bush heavy with blooms. Every plant a different color, deep red, soft white, bright yellow, dark orange, lavender, dark purple, what a show. They looked so different from here, no wonder he liked being Joe Proost, he saw the world through rose-colored glasses.

Alzheimer's patients only see the present, now I saw it too. Joe was only 5'7" but; for me I might as well have been standing on the Empire state building. I felt like I could see for miles. You could tell he was proud of his garden, I could feel his eyes crinkle with a big satisfied grin. In spite of myself, I began to grin too; we were both so happy, so peaceful. His spirit was infiltrating my spirit, it was incredible, we were so blended, and we truly were becoming one. I could have stood there for hours, but the reason I started this journey was close, his brain, I was a little nervous as I headed for the top.

It was a torturous climb, my first impression was clutter, his brain was filled with plaques and tangles, I was afraid of that. I could barely see I had to feel my way around. My face was plastered with sticky, gooey slime; I felt real fear here. I came upon a clearing, ahh! This must be the place where he felt clear. The space was not large but well kept. I felt warm and cozy, I was sure this was the present. Smelling of lavender, that was warm and earthy, it permeated my very fiber. This is the, "in the moment" place, where all Alzheimer's patients live. Here, I could feel what was happening to him now. I could feel his wonder while he was admiring his garden. I could feel him feel my presence; he was not scared; but filled with joy.

When I turned to the left, that was the past, it was dark and gloomy, nothing to see there. The future was to the right, it was covered in a thick fog, Joe, could not see anything here. This place was extremely scary, you cannot move forward if you do not know where you are going, if you do not know what to do next. So I went back to the present, where it was warm and safe, I could feel him here. He was happy, like a young child, full of wonder. The present moment, that is where Joe lived, that is where I lived too.

I began to feel sucked away from Joe, "No, it's too soon," I said, but sadly, my time on the inside had ended. I landed back where I had begun outside, full size. Looking at Joe wander through the roses, I wondered if this was a dream. Did I imagine my recent journey? No, what was that on my face, it was sticky and gooey? I stood very still. My journey had been real.

I left the place that I had wanted to visit, comfortable in the knowledge that Joe, shackled to the earth in a sick body, was happily living in a free and clear space in his mind that housed his true spirit. This was the spirit of a young child living life fully dancing in the present moment. I was happy that I could dance in the moment with him.

When I woke up the next morning, I looked over at Joe; he lay with his head facing mine. The face I had been waking up to each morning looked different now, somehow more peaceful. Every ounce of my being wanted to cry for the love of him; I lay there memorizing his face. I knew that he would not be next to me in bed forever and I wanted to feel this moment.

twenty

"I think we have a problem!"
When you think you have a problem, sing it away.
Wanda

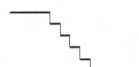

oe was beginning to have trouble sleeping; he would wander around the house at night. Most nights I could feel him get up and I would get up with him. One night, in the middle of winter, Joe got up and I continued sleeping. When I did wake up, he was not in bed with me. I found him in the living room on the couch naked and freezing cold, he was asleep with his arms folded across his chest. It took me a minute to wake him and coax him off the couch; I have never felt so bad. It was a horrible feeling for me. I can only imagine how scared he was.

"Joey, what are you doing out here?"

"I could not find you!" he said.

As a result, I moved our bed so he had to crawl over me to get out, that helped a lot. Although he thought, I was crazy; he looked at me and rolled his eyes. Joe could not find the bathroom since I had moved the bed. No problem, he would crawl off the end of the bed and simply urinate on the carpet in a corner. By solving one problem, I had created another.

Driving with Joe had become a challenge, every time we got about ten minutes away from home he would have to urinate. I could not always find a bathroom. I started taking a jar with me, so he could use it. Sometimes he had to go so bad his aim was off and he would urinate all over the car, another bad idea by Wanda. He was wearing pull on Depends. That helped although he still would try to pull them down. The whole bathroom thing really became a big deal! He would urinate anywhere, in plants in the house, in the closet; I constantly had to watch him. I actually got to the point that when he would drink anything I would cringe!

One night Joe somehow got by me in bed, I think he crawled off the end and went to the bathroom by himself. I was always so tired that sometimes I did not feel him get up. He woke me up with his hands outstretched and filled with his stool.

He looked at me with dismay and said, "We have a problem!"

I said surprised but immediately wide-awake. "Yes, Joe we do have a problem!"

To this day, I laugh about what transpired that night; it was typical of our lives! Yes, we did have a problem! I jumped out of bed, careful not to disturb his outstretched hands, and carefully guided Joe back to the bathroom. There I found stool all over the floor, Joe had stepped in it and it was between his toes and all over the bathroom floor and the bedroom carpet. I tried to get Joe to drop his little package into the toilet, but now he would not let go. After a little coaxing, I finally got him to drop it, missing the toilet.

The immensity of the situation hit me and I began to laugh, Joe looked at me quizzically and he too began to laugh. It was 3am, the only way to clean him up was to take a shower, so we both jumped into the hot running water and thus began another fun filled day in the lives of the Proosts! I was definitely in the moment, I felt everyone.

Cheryl and I laughed and laughed about my late night date with "poop!" To this day, whenever we have something happen, we immediately say, "I think we have a problem!"

These stories, while tragic were very funny, that is what I mean by keeping your sense of humor. If I had cried or gotten mad, Joe would have become scared and the outcome of that day would have been very different. It was the same attitude that got me through wiping him after he had gone to the bathroom, not something I relished. I did not want to embarrass him, and so I would sing while I ministered to him. He got so used to our routine that whenever he would go to the bathroom, he would bend over and immediately start singing!

There have been many stories circulated that show Alzheimer's patients becoming mean, belligerent, and violent. Because my family had heard these stories, they were constantly asking me if Joe was getting violent with me. Joe had always been so sweet and docile that I always answered no. I even became irritated with the attitude that my sweet, loving White Knight could ever stoop to behavior that could put me in jeopardy.

Joe had long sense stopped using my name. He knew he loved me, but forgot who I was, that was so sad for me, but anticipated. When asking for his brother, he would say, my friend.

twenty-one

Sometimes, life becomes so hard, so unbelievable all you can do is scream.
You open your mouth and no sound comes out.
You look at the people around you and silently
ask, "Can't you hear me screaming?"

Wanda

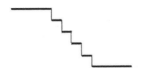

𝒥 sit here praying that I can somehow find the words to convey the sadness and complete devastation of this next saga of our lives. This is about Jim. You cannot fully understand Joe without understanding Jim, as Joe and Jim, being twins and completely devoted to each other affected the way their lives intertwined and finally played out.

Jim's health had begun to deteriorate in the last year; his liver was failing. The sicker Joe got, the sicker Jim got. For Cheryl and me our lives were unbelievable and crazy. Both of our beloved husbands were dying. We really expected Joe to go first; his condition seemed the most tenuous.

Cheryl and I spent almost all of our time now loving and cooking for our two sick husbands. We relied heavily on each other and this was unconditional love. We became one family unit, each feeling the others suffering. Jim was steadfast in his devotion to Joe. He took Joe when I needed a break. Jim would often pick Joe up and take him on small day trips.

Jim rarely complained about the fact that he was in constant pain, choosing to focus on the needs of his beloved brother. Joe was devoted to "his friend" and when in his company could be seen happily following him around whistling. As I live the rest of my life, I do not know if I will ever again see pure unfiltered, unconditional love as demonstrated by those two brothers. Those memories will stand in my memory as a powerful reminder of the true presence of God in our lives. Trying to emulate that love will be a constant measure of my life's goal.

Jim grew sicker and was having trouble walking around the house; his body was becoming weak. He no longer wanted to eat much and was in excruciating pain, but that did not stop us from trying to feed him. Cheryl would come home from work and cook elaborate meals, trying to tempt Jim to eat. She was having great difficulty watching her lifelong love succumb to his illness.

Cheryl was still trying to go to work each day, putting on a brave face, but I could see through her bravado. After working myself in the mornings, Joe and I would spend the afternoons with Jim. We tried valiantly to make him comfortable and I wanted Joe to spend as much time with him as possible. Joe would patiently sit with Jim, sometimes holding his hand, mostly just watching him.

Andon took his dad back to the hospital on the morning, of October 22. Jim was in so much pain that he could barely speak.

"There is nothing more we can do, do you understand, Jim. We are going to send you to comfort care, there we can keep you medicated and comfortable." the doctor said.

As Jim tried to get out of bed, he said, "Take me home, Andon, I want to go home."

Andon brought his dad home at 4pm and Jim died in Cheryl's arms in their home at 7:30pm. There are no words to describe the sadness and the emptiness, but the extreme holiness of that experience. Cheryl stayed with Jim until the funeral parlor arrived, which took over an hour. She kissed him, stroking his face pouring out her love to him, her silent tears falling on his now still chest. I stood there in abject silence watching that holy display of love. A lump rose in my throat and tears stung my eyes as I realized that Jim, my crazy, crazy brother-in-law was gone, and that Joe was next.

I had a lot of trouble trying to figure out how to tell Joe that Jim died; finally, I had no choice. I sat with Joe on our couch and took his hands in mine I looked him straight in his baby blue eyes and said, "Joey, today your friend, Jim died. He loved you so much, he is with God now, and happy."

Joe, just sat there looking at me, he put his head in his hands and did not say a word. I could not tell if he understood me, I had to assume he did. Five minutes later, he was in the refrigerator looking for food.

My mom stayed with Joe for the funeral; she brought him to the party after. Jim loved parties, so we threw him a big one. It was a very chaotic day and Joe was very agitated. Matt and Raechael came for the funeral and that made Joe very happy to have "his people", as he now called them with him that day.

Cheryl, as you can imagine was living a nightmare, kissing and welcoming people to her home all day. Her eyes would well up with tears every time someone came up to her to give their condolences. That night I found her sleeping on the couch clutching Jim's urn in her arms, dried tears on her cheeks.

About three weeks after the funeral Joe and I were in the car going to work and Joe asked. "I want my friend."

I knew "his friend", meant Jim.

"Joey, Jim died, he is in Heaven with God. Jim loved you very much. He is happy now."

Joe looked at me aghast, buried his head in his hands and wept. I was unprepared for his reaction. I pulled our car off to the side of the road, pulled him into my arms, and silently cried with him. My heart broke for Joe.

This time he understood and he stayed focused for a long time. That really moved me; it was the beginning of the end for Joe. We spent a lot of time with Cheryl helping around the house, doing yard work and generally just keeping her company. She had many close friends; that rarely left her side. Joe took two steps down the stairs and now could be see staring off into space most days, I always wondered if he was thinking of Jim.

twenty-two

And God replied, "I am going to answer your prayers. Be vigilant my precious child. I love you, and I will send you many blessings. They will not be what you expect, but what you need. My miracles come in the dark of night when you are your most vulnerable, listen to the wind; it is my whisper to you."

Wanda

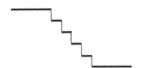

We had had a very busy Saturday, pulling weeds, trimming roses, giving Riley a bath and washing the car. Joe was always happy to help around the house and was in high spirits. I was tired, but happy too.

I said, "Joe would you like me to make you a cake?"

"Yes!" he said, licking his lips.

He stood very close to me as I pulled out the mixer and made our German chocolate cake. This was my favorite cake. Every cake was Joe's favorite, with vanilla ice cream.

As I lovingly finished frosting our cake, I decided we should share it with Brady and Harlyn.

"Hi Harlyn, ask daddy it he would like to come and get some cake, I don't think Joey and I can eat the whole thing." I said through the phone.

I could hear her ask her dad, she came back on the line and said, "Daddy said we'll be right there."

I smiled to myself as I waited for them. The doorbell rang and Joe ran for the door and just stood there waiting for me to open it. Harlyn rushed through the door and into the kitchen to see her cake. Joe followed Harlyn worried about his cake. Brady laughed as he entered the living room; we all headed for the kitchen.

I picked up the knife to cut the cake and Brady said, "Just a small piece."

"Oh, no, Joe and I can't eat a whole cake, I'll give you half.

"Yeah, Granny, half, we'll take half."

"Ok, Harlyn, could you back up a little so I can cut it, you too Joey."

I cut the cake in half, transferring it to another plate. I wrapped it with plastic wrap and Harlyn grabbed it out of my hand. Brady and I laughed as she ran for the door. We followed her and as they started down our front steps, we heard the garbage disposal in the kitchen. Brady and I looked at each other and not seeing Joe ran back to the kitchen.

Joe was standing in front of the sink with the water running. I did not see our half of the cake.

"Joey, where is our cake? What did you do? Did you put our cake down the garbage disposal?"

"Yes, all gone!" He said proudly.

I could not believe it; I really wanted a piece of cake! Harlyn by now was back in the kitchen with her half of the cake. She looked down at her cake and started backing up; she could see the writing on the wall.

Brady said laughing, "Harlyn let's give Granny some of our cake, their cake is gone."

No, daddy, it's mine!"

Brady had to struggle to get the cake out of Harlyn's clutches.

"Here Wanda, cut it in half."

"Yes, cake!" Joe said and tried to grab it from me.

I cut the cake in half again and carried our half to the door with me to see Brady and Harlyn out. Brady laughed all the way to the truck. Harlyn sulked all the way to the truck. Joe ran to the kitchen to get forks. What a night!

I later, thought about Joe and the garbage disposal, he could have put his hand in it and been seriously injured. I never left him in the kitchen alone after that night, another lesson.

Joe began to talk to himself in the mirror. The first day that I noticed this, I was getting ready for work, Joe was dressed waiting for me to put on my make-up and do my hair. I heard voices coming from the other room. I went to see what he was doing and found Joe in the other bathroom talking to the mirror.

I could tell by what he said that he was conducting a business meeting from his old job, where he had been in sales. I was spellbound and intrigued, he sounded just like the old Joe. He held himself with pride and delivered a speech, riddled with gibberish, yet had enough correct language I could follow. Joe actually had me as a captive audience and I could not wait to see what he would say next. This meeting went on for about ten minutes. Finally, he turned around and welcomed me to the meeting, not knowing me; but happy I was there.

I finally excused myself from the meeting, going back to finish getting ready for work. What was this? He ended up conducting meetings whenever he was in front of a mirror, sometimes it would occupy him for half an hour or more. Sometimes Joe would get angry in his meetings; it was then I would steer him to his next snack.

The doctor said that his mirror meetings were very common to Alzheimer's patients. He recommended that I remove or cover all my mirrors. I found this to be unreasonable, so I kept him away from rooms with mirrors when he was agitated.

Sleeping now was more of an issue since Jim's death. Joe would wander around off and on all night long. Sometimes conducting "mirror meetings" in the middle of the night. He was agitated and less cooperative now, taking naps off and on all day. I took him back to the neurologist, who prescribed a sleeping pill. Instead of calming Joe down, they seemed to increase his sleeplessness and agitation. After a few weeks of less than normal sleep, I stopped them. I was more tired than he was, if he did not sleep, neither did I.

Joe's vocabulary had decreased to that of a young child of about two or three. Mostly it was disjointed gibberish, his facial features would contort as a small child's and he would break into a quick grin when given treats. Cookies, candy, cake or his most favorite, iced mocha. It was during these times, I thought of my girls when they were small, the angry outbursts, and the tears, then just as quickly, hugs and kisses and big grins. The two scenarios were hauntingly similar. Joe would tug at my heart; I spent my entire day trying to elicit big grins and loads of hugs.

I was so enmeshed in Alzheimer's, that our "normal" day really did seem normal to me. When someone would say, "I do not know how you do It." or "You are a saint, I could never take care of my husband the way you take care of Joe", I honestly could not see myself doing anything extraordinary. Our life was extraordinary, not me. I was really just an observer to Joe's amazing journey. I knew I was party to one of God's most amazing miracles. I felt thankful that I could be there to witness the unbelievable events that were enveloping Joe. Joe kept me mesmerized as he began to transition from this life to the next. I began to cover him with the cloak of love. I now was his White Knight permanently.

Every night, I would pray for Joe. It was hard to know exactly how to phrase my prayers. If I prayed for this to be over, Joe would be gone. Even though, I was really becoming tired of watching Joe struggle, I could not imagine my life without him. So, I prayed for peace and the wisdom to know what to do next for both of us. I prayed for Joe to suddenly sit up one day and tell me he loved me, hug me and kiss me and call me by my name. I knew this was an unrealistic prayer and I knew Joe had to walk his own path. The love I felt for him offered me no choice, sometimes when we feel such a strong love we fall prey to false hope. Sometimes that hope shines, even if just for a moment.

twenty-three

Violence came like a thief in the night.

Unchecked, it threatened to topple our precarious world.

Our days were numbered; it obliterated the light.

My love came in waves, like a flag unfurled.

Wanda

*J*oe got up to use the bathroom in the middle of the night, I got up with him, he was very nervous, and I was extremely tired. When I tried to get him back in bed, he refused. I asked him a second time and without warning, he pushed me on the bed, jumped on top of me, and pinned my arms over my head. Joe was much stronger than I was and had boxed in school. When I struggled under his weigh, he became stronger and angrier.

Joe made a fist and cocked his arm back as if he was going to punch me, I yelled, "Joe I'm your wife, Wanda, don't hit me Joey. Please Joey please don't hit me, I'm Wanda, I'm your wife, you love me!"

My mind was racing, I felt for the first time, real fear. I was in mortal danger and from the man I loved the most. It was 2am and I was alone. Joe sat on top of me for what seemed like for-ever, then slowly lowered his arm, unclenched his fist, and rolled off me. It was at that moment that I realized I needed help. Our lives changed that night forever.

I sat with Joe calming him down, talking softly to him; stroking his hair. He finally kissed me rolled over and promptly fell asleep. I lay awake all night, my mind racing. I did not know what to do now.

The next day Cheryl came over for a visit, she was still reeling from Jim's death and just wanted to talk. I promised myself that I would not tell anyone about Joe's physical outburst, however as Cheryl and I began to pour out our troubles to each other, it just slipped out. Cheryl was outraged and scared for me.

Cheryl said, "You've done enough! This is over! Wanda, you have to put him in a convalescent hospital. He's going to hurt you and I will not stand for that. You've done all you can, now you have to let others take care of him. He doesn't even know you anymore."

I started to cry and asked, "If Jim was here, what would he tell me to do?"

Cheryl, now also in tears said, "Jim would tell you the same thing, you've done all you can, Joe is a danger to you. Wanda this is bigger than you, and I won't let you do this anymore!"

We sat for a long time holding each other, both crying for our husbands, for ourselves, our lives were out of control; we were lost in pain and fear. Sobs racked my body, deep unrelenting sobs that came up from deep in my soul.

I knew Cheryl was right. I had promised Joe that I would stay with him forever, now I was going to break that promise. I was weary, so weary that I could not think.

Cheryl pressed me, "I mean it, Wanda I want you to get help right away, promise me!"

I slowly said, "Yes I promise I'll check into a convalescent hospital."

I tiptoed around Joe all day, afraid I would somehow make him angry again. That night before I went to bed I put all the kitchen knives away under the sink behind the garbage can. I really did not know what Joe was now capable of, but I was scared. I did not sleep very well even though Joe slept and nothing abnormal happened. A couple of days went by and I began to notice Joe less cooperative with me.

Joe refused to get in the car to go to work two days later. I had to call my client and cancel my housecleaning with her. I lied and said Joe had the flu; I did not want to admit that he was becoming uncooperative. I was afraid to say those words aloud; it would make it more real somehow.

Everyone had warned me this might happen and I had always said, "No, Joe would not become violent; he was too easygoing." I was wrong.

Once, I got used to the idea that I could no longer keep Joe with me; I got busy. The first thing I needed to do was sign him up for Medi-cal. I could not afford to pay for convalescent care, which ran about $4,000.00 to $5,000.00 a month. This task is not for the faint of heart, long lines at the Medi-cal office, two appointments, piles of paperwork and all of our supporting paperwork, and tons of patience. I was a little low on patience. It took about three weeks to get him approved.

In the evenings, while Joe would nap on the couch, I would hold his hand and watch him. I knew in my heart that my time with him was short. I memorized his face, the way his hands would rest on his chest, the lines of his once strong square jaw. I would talk to God and ask him to bless this beautiful man, and I would thank him for the privilege of being Joe's wife. Joe had been my White Knight in Shining Armor. Now, his armor had faded away, but he was still my Knight. I had become his armor, ready to do battle at the first hint of trouble; I threw my love around him like a cloak.

As soon as I got his Medi-cal card in the mail, I jumped on the phone to find a convalescent hospital that would take his insurance and could accommodate the fact that he was a wanderer. There were no facilities in Santa Cruz County that could take Joe. I was frantic; he was becoming more uncooperative and harder to control. I was sometimes afraid of him. I started calling in Monterey County, they were either full or did not have the accommodations we needed. Finally, near tears, I dialed the last number on my list, they had one bed left, and I took it sight unseen. I made an appointment to visit the convalescent hospital the next day. I took my mom with us. I was so nervous that I could hardly drive.

The tape in my head ran like this; "What am I doing? Am I abandoning my responsibility, am I a quitter? Do I have the right to leave Joe just because he is getting harder to control? Will I be able to live with this decision? Will he be lonely, what if he has a lucid moment and I am not with him, will he be scared? What if he hurts someone, am I a bad wife? What about the promise I made him?"

My mom kept telling me, that I was doing the right thing for both of us. This disease affects the whole family; I know that it killed my mom to have to watch me with Joe. She hated to see me work so hard. Mom always kept a brave face for me, while I was doing the same thing for her. We both knew it but kept up the façade; it was what kept us going.

twenty-four

When you make a commitment to love someone 'til death do you
part; you seldom expect to part mentally while they are still alive.
Love cannot always shield your heart.
As you look back sometime later, you will know with
certainty that your love was worth it.

Wanda

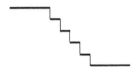

J smiled through my tears as we entered Joe's new home. The facility was big, thirty-two Alzheimer's patients in the locked section of the convalescent hospital and another larger wing with patients in various stages of sickness and just plain age. The lobby had a huge fish tank and an aviary outside, it was clean and beautiful, and the staff was concerned and dedicated. They were committed to making both Joe and me as comfortable as possible. I breathed a sigh of relief, the last bed and in such a beautiful place. I spent a lot of time saying thank you to God; he was with me every step of the way.

There was a problem; I had to transfer Joe's Medi-cal from Santa Cruz County to Monterey County. It took almost two months. They admitted him, but I had to pay a deposit up front. I had another choice now. Pay my mortgage or pay the convalescent hospital, I could not afford both. The day after Joe's sixty-second birthday, I admitted him. I knew I was going to lose our house; nothing compared to losing my husband!

Joe's Birthday was bitter sweet; it was my last full day with him alone in our home. Each moment was precious; I remember every moment of love, every look, every touch, I remember the essence of him. I baked him a German chocolate cake. We sat at the coffee table watching a movie and with two forks ate it right off the plate. We used to do that when he was healthy, it was kind of bohemian, but fun! Joe dove in; he loved cake, I could barely swallow mine.

When we went to bed that night, Joe put his arm around me and fell into a deep sleep. I laid my head on his chest, as I had so many times before. I could not stop the silent tears that rolled onto his chest; I did not try to wipe them away. Sleep for me was elusive; I reveled in the feeling of his ever so slightly hairy chest, his breath on my hair.

I prayed for both of us that night, peace for Joe and forgiveness for me. I felt like I had somehow fallen short and I had let Joe down. I remember thinking that knowing and loving Joe had been the best gift ever. The gift of love like no other; I really did see God when I looked into his eyes. Our marriage was so short, ten years, but they were jam packed with love every day. It had been an honor and a privilege to love Joe.

Joe and I had to clean a house in the morning before I took him to the convalescent hospital. I was so distracted that I do not remember cleaning that morning. Joe spent the morning sleeping in my client's recliner. Sometimes, I would stop and just watch him sleep, knowing this was the last time I would get to watch him uninterrupted. I took snap shots of him in my mind, to bring them out later when I was alone.

Time slowed to a crawl as we drove to his new home. I had not told Joe that he was not going to live with me anymore because I knew he would just forget and I was worried that he would get scared.

While we were driving to the convalescent hospital I told him," Joey, remember when we went to visit the home with all the people?"

He shook his head, "Yes."

I knew he did not, "Well, they need help with some of the people that live there, things that you can do for them, like folding clothes, visiting and keeping some of them company. You are going to stay with the people and help them."

He looked at me with childlike wonder. "I want you."

"I'll come to be with you every day."

He held my hand and began to sing with the radio that was playing in the car. I thought I was going to throw up, my heart was breaking and I could not cry. I swallowed the large lump in my throat and blinked back stinging tears. For a while, I could not speak; content to listen to Joe sing off key and happy to feel him stroking the inside of my right wrist.

When we got to the convalescent hospital, I grabbed Joe's suitcase and helped him out of the car. He hugged me long and hard.

"I love you!" he said.

"I love you too, Joey, you're going to be all right. No one could have had a more wonderful husband, thank you for being my White Knight, now let's go and meet all of your new friends."

I walked into the admissions office with Joe dutifully walking behind me; he had a tight grip on my hand. The admissions coordinator showed us to two comfortable brown leather chairs. I took a deep breath as she introduced herself and handed me a very large packet of information. I grabbed a pen out of my purse and set about filling out all the information required. Joe sat in his chair and was very quiet. I could not tell if he knew what was happening but I was hesitant to ask too many questions with him there.

After about ten minutes, a nurse came into the office to take Joe back to his locked wing, she asked him to go with her. She put out her hand and Joe stood up took her hand and let himself be led away with her. As he went through the doorway, he turned to look back at me.

"Go ahead Joey, I'll be there in a minute, go meet your new friends; they need you."

He nodded, smiled, and walked out. After they were gone, the tears that were stinging my eyes slowly trickled down my face. I finally found my voice.

"I am so thankful that you had a bed for Joe, I'm nervous to leave him, he's been with me day and night for the last few years, and I'm worried that he'll think I've abandoned him."

She answered in a kind and loving voice, "Don't worry about Joe, we'll take very good care of him. Our doctor on staff will examine him and we will monitor his behavior to be sure he is comfortable with his new surroundings. Patients generally do quite well. He will probably have some adjustments, but will enjoy the interaction of patients just like him."

She continued, "Joe is the youngest patient we have and will get a lot of attention from our nursing staff. We'll make sure that he's comfortable."

"Thank you, that makes me feel a little better." I choked.

"We have to talk about a sensitive subject, the DNR, do not resuscitate form." She became very serious as she handed it to me. I read it and began to fill it out.

"Have you thought about a DNR?"

"Yes, Joe and I talked about this when we first got married; he told me that if anything bad ever happened to him, he would not want to be resuscitated."

I signed and dated Joe's DNR and handed it back to her along with my power of attorney and his living will.

"I'm impressed that you're so prepared, most caregivers are not, you wouldn't believe the amount of people that refuse to sign a DNR"

"Joe has Alzheimer's and will never get better, why would I resuscitate him to continue living an Alzheimer's life in a convalescent hospital. I have thought long and hard about this, it's the only fair thing to do for Joe. It's because I love him that I sign this form. Make no mistake I'm saddened beyond all belief that this disease has brought me to this decision. I know that you'll do everything possible to make him as comfortable as you can, that's why I'm leaving him here with you."

I got up to leave, she came up to me and gave me a hug and said, "You're very brave, Joe is lucky to have you."

"I'm the lucky one, Joe has been the most amazing man and husband; he would have done this for me. It's so weird, I miss him already."

"I know sweetheart, I know." She started to cry.

I caught up with Joe and took him to his room, which he shared with two other male patients. He held my hand tightly as I showed him his bed and his closet. I could not believe that our life together had come to this, a twin bed, shared closet and a bathroom. Joe's identity was gone. Unless, you have experienced this with a loved one, there are no words to describe the unbelievable agony of that day.

On the other hand, thankfully Joe did not remember his past life with me. He did not view his situation as dire, only confusing. Joe had no idea who I was or what we had meant to each other and he did not know my name.

The week before his admission, I began to prepare. I bought him seven pairs of pajamas, seven pairs of sweats, two pairs of slippers, seven long sleeve t-shirts and seven pairs of socks and underwear. I did not want him to look like the rest of the population in convalescent hospitals unkempt with clothes that did not fit or match. I carefully labeled each piece of clothing with his name. Naive of me for sure, but I loved him so much that I wanted him to be in his own comfortable clothes. It was important to me that he maintained at least some of his dignity. I loving unpacked his suitcase and put his meager belongings away. I put two pictures on his nightstand, one of me and one of him with his baby grandson Elijah.

I took Joe to the great room; there the residents ate and associated with each other. They were in varying stages of dementia, some sat in wheel chairs drooling, other wandered aimlessly and still others sat and cried. I sat down with Joe as he became acquainted with his surroundings. Finally, I could not take another minute, I had to leave; I had to get out of there.

I took Joe in my arms and whispered in his ear," I love you so much, be good and help the people, I'll be back very soon to see you."

Joe did not answer; he had gone to his special place, a place I could not go. He sat down with one of the female residents and grabbed her hand as he began to talk to her. I walked out, and my heart was broken.

As I walked past the office, the manager stopped me and said, "Please don't come see Joe for ten days; we need to get him used to us. If you see him too soon, he may want to go home; it will hurt him more than help him."

I had not thought of that, I started to argue with her; however, I knew that in my heart she was right.

"Ok, will you call me if you have any questions, or if anything goes wrong. Can I call the nurses each day to inquire how he's doing?"

"Yes, feel free to call we'll update you on his condition every day."

I did not see that coming, I really felt like I had just abandoned him. My steps to the car slowed; my feet leaden. Tears were building behind my eyes, which threatened to explode like a dam bursting. As I shut the car door, I screamed, a deep animal sound that came from a deep, dark place inside of me. Then, I sobbed, after a few minutes I pulled the car out of the parking lot to go home, alone.

twenty-five

Moments of intense joy and intense pain are burned in your memory forever.
Both emotions happen at the same time with caregivers.
Caregivers call this Alzheimer's.

Wanda

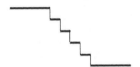

Have you ever noticed that when you are happy time speeds up and when you are sad how slow time moves? Today time stopped for me. I drove home alone, my mind racing, the relief everyone said I would feel did not come, only emptiness and silence. The lump in my throat threatened to stop my breathing. Joe's journey home began today; I would not be a part of his last days on this earth. There would only be fleeting moments that would be the most painful I had ever experienced.

As I lay in my cold empty bed that first night, I thought about how my life had unfolded since Joe's illness. I remembered the tender, funny moments we had shared. The loving and intelligent man he once was.

I began to pray and this was my prayer.

"Dear God, please take Joe out of that convalescent hospital, please just take him as fast as possible. Please don't let him die a slow Alzheimer's death, get him out of there!"

I prayed that prayer every night until he died!

I went to work the next day and every day after that. My family tried everything to give me as normal a life as possible. Someone was always popping over; Cheryl had become my constant companion when I was not working. We spent a lot of time crying over our husbands, Jim gone now and Joe in limbo. We also spent a lot of time laughing and reminiscing over our lives and the loving and sometimes infuriating things our husbands had done. Cheryl and I told the same stories to each other over and over; it helped somehow.

I waited impatiently for the first ten days to pass until I could see Joe. Nothing could have prepared me for what I found. A nurse buzzed me through the locked double doors. My heart was in my throat as patients wandering aimlessly up and down the long stark corridor, their faces devoid of emotion. I walked to the end and into the great room, Joe was sitting next to the same woman that he was holding hands with when I left him last.

Joe was chatting with her and holding her hand. He did not see me approach, as I got closer I said, "Hi Joey, do you remember me?"

He looked at me not knowing who I was, I sat down next to him, he turned to me and smiled, shifted his body to face me and said," Hi, my friend."

For a moment he knew me; he grabbed my hand and I said," Let's go for a walk."

We walked hand in hand through the locked door out to the sparsely planted garden. We sat at a round picnic table with no umbrella; it was so depressing. I offered Joe the mocha I had brought him; he did not know what it was. I showed him how to suck out of the straw; he took a couple of sips and put it down, not his favorite drink anymore.

Joe was wearing someone else's shirt and pants, they did not fit well, he had on his slippers with no socks. His feet felt cold, so I took off my socks and put them on him. I made a mental note to go through his closet before I left to see if he still had any of his clothes. Joe looked just like all the rest of the patients, clean, but unkempt. My worst fear realized; my Joe was gone.

Joe did not make eye contact with me; instead, his eyes would dart around not focusing on any one thing. He continued to hold my hand, but it did not feel the same to me, there was no feeling in Joe so his hand was lifeless. His skin that was once ruddy and full of life, was now pale and pasty looking. This was not my husband, he even looked older and very different somehow, I had to get used to that. I cannot really describe was I was feeling. The longer I sat there talking to him, the more I wanted to run.

Finally, I could take it no longer and took Joe back to the great room. I sat him back with the same woman he had been holding hands with before and he immediately became very animated and grabbed for her hand. She let him take it and I turned away, wiping tears from my eyes. It was done, he was gone and in his place a stranger and in my heart a hole.

I went to see Joe almost every day, sometimes I would take my Mom and sometimes Cheryl. It was easier to be alone though, because when I was with someone I had to pretend to be ok. I was not and being alone was less stressful. Every time I saw Joe, he looked worse, he now had hair growing out of his ears and nose and his hair was getting long. His nails, while clean were too long. Joe was always fastidious about his grooming and would have been appalled at the way he looked. The nurses said that he had refused to let them groom him. Per their protocol; they step away and do not force their patients to do anything.

This was a living nightmare and Joe was the main character, I had a supporting role. Almost like watching a horror movie play out right before my eyes. All of Joe's clothes had been misplaced; I checked they were not even in the building. He was wearing other patients clothes mismatched and misfit. Joe's favorite pillow, handmade blanket and his Tilley hat; all were gone. Just like Joe, gone. I could barely stand to walk into the convalescent hospital, yet I could not wait to get there!

While I was visiting one day, Joe said he had to go to the bathroom. I walked him to his room, which had an attached bathroom. He let me help him out of his diaper and while he was standing over the toilet relieving him; he looked over at me and unexpectedly said, "You know, Wanda everyone out there is crazy!"

I laughed and said, "I know Joey, I know!"

Our eyes met and just for an instant, we were back in our bathroom laughing over something silly. That small exchange was such a gift for me and my heart was full.

I said, "I love you."

Joe said, "I love you too."

Then he was gone, eyes vacant not really seeing me anymore.

Most visits were like that, for a moment when we would look at each other and we would connect, Joe would know me. Sometimes it was just a squeeze of his hand, or a knowing grin. Sometimes, I would get a kiss or a quick hug. Then off again into his private world, a world that I could not share with him. I missed my husband dearly.

The nurses told me Joe had stopped dancing, and had become more frantic. Whenever he heard music, he danced, mostly alone sometimes with the nurses. One day, while I was visiting a nurse put on some music. Joe looked at me, took my hand, and led me to the middle of the floor. We danced as we had done so many times before. I closed my eyes and rested my head on his shoulder. Silent tears streamed down my face, this disease was so unfair; I wanted my husband back.

"I pleaded with God; please give me back my husband!"

It occurred to me that Joe was between two worlds. He was neither here, nor there, not dead but certainly not alive. This was where Joe lived and I lived there too. Could it be that we had been too happy with each other? I doubted that, we were born to be happy. I began to read everything I could get my hands on that pertained to death and dying and the afterlife. I had plenty of time at night alone in my empty house. It had ceased to be a home the day Joe had left, now it was just a place to sleep and rarely eat. I was suffering watching Joe suffer. I felt like I was dying with him.

Then one day I was listening to a tape in the car by a Doctor and public speaker, he said, "Alzheimer's patients are closer to

God than the rest of us, they are like little children, pure and innocent."

I felt so much better; at least God was with Joe, because God was with all the innocent children.

He went on to say, "When someone you love dies, there is a hole in your heart that God fills with his Grace." I prayed that God would fill the hole in my heart with Grace and peace.

Sometimes when Joe used to talk to himself I could not always understand him, yet he carried on what seemed like a real conversation, I believe he was talking to God, or his angel, or spirit guide. I believe now, that Joe was preparing himself to go home.

It was exactly seventy-nine days since Joe's admittance to the hospital. I do not know why but that morning I had counted the days. I was surprised how fast and how slow the time had gone. Today I was taking my mom and Cheryl with me. We had never all gone together, but for some reason I wanted them both with me. I had a bad feeling about today; the hairs were standing up on my arms. I felt scared, more than usual and did not want to be alone; I could barely breathe.

We arrived at the convalescent hospital about 1pm. Lunch was over and the residents were wandering around the halls and the great room. Nothing could have prepared me for what I saw. Joe was on his hands and knees, no shirt and no shoes, his hair was long and eschew. He was frantically scratching the floor with both hands. He looked like a wild man. All three of us stood there with our mouths open, the nurses in the room acted as if they did not see Joe until I rushed up to him trying to get him off the floor.

"Joey, it's me, its Wanda your wife, get up Joey!"

Joe did not look at me; he just kept scratching the floor, as if he was trying to dig his way out! Finally, one of the nurses came over and helped me with Joe, another one ran over with his shirt. I had to turn it right side out before I could put it on him, which was a struggle. We found his slippers and I grabbed his hand and took him out of the great room.

"Joey, would you like to go for a walk with me?"

He looked at me with those blank, distant eyes.

"Come on Joe, let's go for a walk."

He let me lead him out towards the lobby. My mom and Cheryl followed behind us, silent heads bowed. We took him into the lobby where the fish tank was, I tried to get him interested in the fish to no avail. I was so upset that I finally took him over to one of the couches and sat down with him still holding his hand.

I spoke to him softly, as I stroked his hand. "How are you, Joey? Do you remember me, I am Wanda; your wife."

Joe did not make eye contact with me, his eyes were darting all over the room, and he was very agitated. He began to speak to me and became very animated; I could not understand him. I talked to Joe about his children assuring him that everyone was fine.

He kept on with his gibberish when all of a sudden I heard him say Matt.

"Matt, is good Joe, he misses you so much, are you missing him Joe?"

Joe looked at me and for just a moment, I could see him. Then he was gone, eyes blank.

My mom and Cheryl were across the room watching us, I know that they were scared; but they did not say anything. They tried to act as if this was just a normal visit, but it was not. Joe was wired and crazy. His eyes were darting all around the room it was as if he was trying to escape his own skin. Finally, after an hour we all had had enough, I told Joe that we should go back. He let me lead him past the locked doors to his wing of the hospital.

When the doors slammed behind us, Joe turned to me and put his hands on my face, looked me straight in the eyes and said, "My dear wife you are so beautiful, I love you so much." Then he kissed me, long and slow. He stepped away from me, still holding my face.

I whispered back," I love you so much Joe; you have been the love of my life, you have been my White Knight in Shining Armor, no one could have had a better husband. I think you are beautiful too, thank you for loving me!"

He took me in his arms and gave me a full body hug and then he was gone, eyes darting all around.

Joe stopped looking at me and I knew he had gone back to his special place. I led him back to the great room, sat him next to his woman friend. He grabbed her hand; I stood there for a long time watching him, tears streaming down my cheeks unchecked.

Finally, with a very heavy heart I left. Something was different today; this was not a normal visit for us. My mom and Cheryl had gone outside to wait for me by the car. We decided to go shopping, I was killing time and I did not know why. We drove there in silence as the afternoons events weighed heavily on our minds.

The three of us wandered aimlessly around the store for half an hour. I was the only one loading the shopping cart with items I did not need. Suddenly, I was startled by my cell phone ringing; it was the nurse at the convalescent hospital.

"Mrs. Proost, Joe has collapsed, we think he has had a seizure, he is foaming at the mouth. The fire department and EMT's are standing over him. I know you have signed a do not resuscitate form, but I have to ask you, do you want us to resuscitate?"

Time stopped for me, "What?" I said.

She repeated her question. I grabbed Cheryl's hand and in a very loud voice I said, "No, do not resuscitate!"

"I signed a DNR!" I yelled at her.

The poor nurse on the other end of the phone said, "I'm sorry we needed you to say it."

Again, I said, "DO NOT resuscitate!"

She said, "Ok, meet us at the Hospital, which was just a couple of blocks away from the convalescent hospital, we are taking him there."

"Ok!"

"Oh my God, Cheryl, I just killed him!"

"No, you did not!" she cried, shaking her head.

I had to stop myself from running out of the store, but I was walking very fast. Cheryl and my mom were following mostly in shock. My head was buzzing and my mouth was dry as I reached my car.

My mom said, "You shouldn't drive but Cheryl and I can't drive a stick shift!"

"That's ok, I can drive, hurry, get in! Oh, God mom is this really happening?"

My lips were stiff, I could barely speak; my heart was racing in my chest. I could not believe this was happening so soon. As I merged onto the highway, my cell phone rang again.

The nurse said, "Mrs. Proost don't go to the Hospital."

I said, "Why not?"

"Just come to the convalescent hospital."

Again, I said, "Why not?"

She hesitated for a minute, and then said," I'd rather not say on the phone."

I was really getting frustrated with her!

"Tell me, what happened, please!" I begged.

Finally, in a slow sad voice she said, "Your husband died."

"What, he died?"

"Yes, he was dead in four minutes, we could not have revived him; he had a massive heart attack."

Cheryl from the back seat said, "He died?"

"Yes!" I barely choked out.

This was so surreal; I was driving on autopilot. My mom put her hand on my arm, and said, "This is for the best, it's good for Joe."

"I know." I whispered.

I kept thinking how lucky that I could say good-by to him, and that he knew me one last time. I was also so grateful that I did not have to watch him die. At least I would not have that awful sight playing in my head for the rest of my life. I missed it by thirty minutes; I wondered if Joe knew and that is why he said all those beautiful things to me, he had been telling me good-bye.

We were only a few minutes away, as we pulled into the parking lot, the fire department and the ambulance were there motors running. People were milling around wondering, what had happened. I jumped out of the car and ran into the locked ward, past the nurses' station and into the great room. There on the floor covered by a sheet was Joe. My mouth was dry, I could not swallow, and I could not breathe. Joe's left wrist and right foot were exposed. I stood over him frozen and in complete disbelief.

One of the nurses rushed up to me, grabbed my shoulders and tried to usher me out of the room. I could not move.

I had tried to imagine what this moment would be like, however I could not have imagined this.

She finally said, "Come on, you don't need to see this we will clean him up, you can see him later."

I let her lead me away to the nurses' station. The first thing I did was to call Raechael and Matt.

I took a deep breath as I dialed their number, I did not know how to tell them, and I started to cry as Raechael answered. "Hello."

"Raechael, it's Wanda, Joe just died!"

"What, he died?" She broke into tears.

"Where are you?" she asked.

"At the convalescent hospital, I was here earlier and thirty minutes after I left they called me to come back."

We were both crying we could barely speak, "I'll call you later this evening, I have to go now, the nurses want to talk to me."

"Are you ok, Wanda?"

"Yes, no, I will be, Cheryl and my mom are with me, I love you, go be with Matt, I will call you later."

All of the nurses gathered around me asking if I was all right, I kept saying, "yes", but how could anyone be all right?

Finally the nurse that spent the most time with Joe came to me and said," Joe stopped dancing a couple of weeks after he got here. Today after you left, we put on music and he began dancing all by himself. He had his arms stretched out as if he was dancing with someone. Then, all of a sudden, he groaned and fell. By the time the ambulance got here he was gone."

I will always believe Joe was dancing with his brother Jim. Joe danced his way into Heaven.

After filling out many forms, and calling the mortuary to pick up Joe, a nurse came up to me and said, "Your husband is ready if you would like to see him, he's in the last room on the right."

I said, "No, thank you, I don't want to see him like this, I prefer to remember him the way he was."

With a shocked look on her face, she asked again, "You do not want to see your husband?"

I said in a tired voice barely audible, "No!"

With that, I turned on my heels and left for the last time.

My mom and Cheryl stayed outside by the car as I took off running into the convalescent hospital, now as I approached them I could tell they were at a loss for words.

Mom cradled me in her arms, rocking me back and forth. "Oh, Wanda I'm so sorry, this is for the best. For Joe this is a blessing, you didn't want him to suffer anymore."

"I know you're right, mom I'm so happy for Joe, I just didn't expect him to die like this." I was having trouble breathing.

Cheryl stood there opened her arms and enveloped my limp body. I put my head on her shoulder and as she stroked my hair, she whispered in my ear. "Joe is with Jim now. You'll be all right, we'll be all right." I shook my head yes and sobbed.

"I know!" I choked, "I'm just shocked that he's actually gone, I don't know what I was expecting, but this feels unreal to me."

"I prayed to God to take Joe home, but I did not think it would happen so fast!"

"If you ask me to pray for something, be sure you really want it, because you'll get it!"

With that we all laughed, I wiped tears from my eyes as I got in the car to drive us home for the last time.

The day for most people was just a normal day but for me everything looked and felt different, I was now a widow. I was alone at the bottom of the stairs of life. The sky and the earth felt different somehow. I felt like I was in suspended animation. Driving home on autopilot all I could think about was Joe, and where he had gone. Was he really in Heaven with God; was he really with Jim? My mind was racing, while my body felt still.

"I can't believe Joe is dead!" I said repeatedly all the way home.

Phone calls and cards from friends and family filled my next two weeks. Cheryl and my mom barely left my side. Cheryl moved in with me so I would not be alone. We spent hours reminiscing about Jim and Joe, laughing and crying. My family watched me very closely. My girls were either with me or on the phone with me.

We gave Joe a beautiful memorial party, everyone that loved us came. Family and friends brought food and flowers. We celebrated the wonderful man he was, I walked through the day as if in a dream, my wonderful love affair was over. I felt so empty. I could not feel my feet. Joe's work upon this earth was finished; he had gone home.

The beginning of this book refers to a White Knight; Joe was that Knight for me. Our love felt like a fairy tale and romance novel all in one. Joe and I knew from the beginning that our days were extraordinary, that each moment was precious and we cherished every one of them. We lived a lifetime in ten short years moment by moment.

twenty-six

Every life on this earth affects every other life.
We are all one, clothed in different bodies, living separate lives.
What unites us is unconditional love.

Wanda

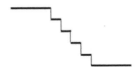

I want to remind you, the reader that I am not a nurse, or professional caregiver, or a physiologist. I am just a regular homemaker, mother and grandmother. I would like to take this opportunity to give you my humble views that are very important to me. Maybe, they will resonate with some of you.

When Joe died, I stood alone at the bottom of our stairs, it took me three years to "wake up". The "wake up" has come in the form of our story. There are so many people with the diagnosis of Alzheimer's and at least an equal number of caregivers. Most come in the form of close family, wives, and husbands. There are also many professional caregivers taking very good care of patients that they have come to know only through this disease.

Alzheimer's is insidious; it does not show favor. People from all occupations, rich and poor, educated and uneducated are affected. When you least expect it, your world can be turned upside down with this diagnosis. Most loved ones step up to the plate, rise to the occasion and do what is necessary. All have broken hearts, many have broken spirits and some never fully recover. There is no manual to tell you what to do, or how to take care of your loved one or patient. That would be like asking God for a manual to come with a newborn baby.

There are books that describe this disease, how the unraveling process works. You will read about plaques and tangles in the brain. Each person is unique; there are no definitive answers on how to parent backwards. Watching someone that was a grown up slide backward in time right before your eyes is daunting. One minute you are in the prime of your life, the next you are a caregiver for someone that has become a young child.

I am not a saint; there were days when I would lose my patience. Sometimes I would dream of jumping on a train going anywhere, because I was so tired. Crying myself to sleep at night, I would ask myself what I could do better. This reminded me of raising my young children. There is a parallel here.

I also realize that there are caregivers who will scoff at my account; that it is too idealistic, too romanticized, I understand. However, this was our life and we lived it. My intent in writing this book is to introduce the idea of staying in the moment with your loved one or patient. I want all caregivers to realize that their attitude directly affects their patients or loved ones. This attitude will help you, the caregiver. In helping, yourself to see this disease in a different light you will inadvertently help your patient stay calm and happy and make both of your lives more enjoyable and sustainable.

Alzheimer's disease reminds me of a staircase. Have you ever watched a baby climb stairs for the first time? They take one-step at a time, wait look to see if anyone is watching, then maybe another. After a while, they are climbing up two steps at a time and so on. Alzheimer's patients walk down the stairs and do not look to see if anyone is watching. First, they go down one-step, they may wait a while then go down another. Then two at a time, sometimes they slip three steps down and you panic that they may fall all the way down. You put out your hand to catch them.

Caregivers are there holding their hands, helping them down the stairs of life.

Caregivers never know when their patient may take another step down, and that is where the terror lies. Fear of the unknown is a powerful force and no laughing matter. The laughing comes, when you can stay in the moment, really feel the moment with your loved one, and realize that living this way comes with its own rewards. I will always remember all of the funny times and the sad times. Laughing just made us feel better and our lives easier. Singing also helps, it is a calming balm on a stinging wound.

Staying in the moment seemed to be the key to my success as a caregiver/mother. As long as I did not compare Joe to his previous healthy self, I was ok. The tears only came when I was tired and I remembered him as he was, or anticipated a very uncertain oblique future.

Joe taught me a great lesson.

Love is everything, love can be fleeting, each day is precious, do not waste them. When you love someone, tell him or her often. Love them unconditionally, no matter what. No one ever gets tired of hearing those three little words. I love you. They buoy you up they lift your soul.

Here is what you can do:

Give to the Alzheimer's Foundation of America. They have already done all the work for you, they have an amazing organization and can give you numerous ways to help. They are a tremendous support for caregivers. We need them.

If you know someone affected with this disease, treat them just like a "normal' person, their caregivers will appreciate that. For as long as possible involve them in family parties, events and do not forget vacations. Everything you do for the patient you do for the caregiver. Believe me the caregiver needs more help than the patient!

As far as the caregivers, give them all your love and support, try shopping or gardening for them. Errands with an Alzheimer's patient are like taking a three year old with you, it can be exhausting. Step in for them as much as possible, even when a caregiver says, no. They do not mean it, most of the time they are too scared to ask. Remember the hugs, they may not get them anymore, everyone needs physical contact.

Let them vent without judgment, or cry and remember to let them laugh. These patients can be very funny. You do not want a caregiver to feel guilty for laughing at something a patient may have done or said. Remember Joe seeing me naked for the first time, he was hilarious and yes, I did laugh!

No matter what religious affiliation you may have, whether you are spiritual or do not believe in "God" remember, there is a higher power. Give yourself over to it; pray if you can; miracles will happen. Joe and I are living proof. I have been witness to many miracles.

As Joe once said to me, "Watch the signs."

Be vigilant, every day is a blessing, it may be that you will be a miracle in someone's life. What a privilege that is, I believe God works through us to perform his many miracles; it is a humbling experience!

Good bye my darling Joe, I wish you safe travel. I can sometimes feel you in a song we once shared, or in the words of a friend. I can feel you; in the early morning "first light" and when I go to the "Big Lake" (ocean). I see you in your children and Elijah. Mostly when I am in the car, we sang songs and laughed in the car. You would hold my hand as I drove. Goodbye my White Knight, until we meet again.

I will spend the rest of my life spreading your peace and love to everyone in the land.

As with all fairy tales, the last line is:

THE END

Epilogue

"And now it's time for me to climb back up the stairs,
one step at a time, moment by moment."
Wanda

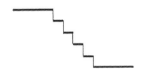

When Joe died, I suddenly found myself at the bottom of the stairs we had so consciously climbed down together moment by moment. I was stupefied to see myself there alone. My despair and deep sadness permeated my every breath. I looked up at the stairs, they seemed so steep and where they would lead, I did not know. I knew I would have to climb them one at a time until I reached the top. I would have to do this alone. Surrounded by family and close friends; the hard work of reaching the top was my burden and mine alone. My emotions ran the gamut, scared, sad, happy for Joe, angry and mostly lost. I did not think I could exist in this world without him.

Emotionally I had shut down. In order to remain sane; I had closed off my feelings and went about my daily tasks like a wooden soldier. It took me a long time to gather the courage to put my foot on that first stair. Slowly I began to climb up the stairs that Joe and I had traveled down together. It took Joe four years to reach the bottom and it took four long years for me to reach the top.

Along the way, I stumbled and sometimes cried out for him in the darkness of the lonely nights. I knew he was with me, I could feel him, when I least expected it. I drew strength from our boundless love and abiding joy in the ordinary moments of our lives together. I had a problem; I could not seem to stay in that feeling for long.

Those first few steps were hard, I felt numb, the world seemed hazy to me. I had forgotten the lessons learned from Joe. One night I cried out for him to help me, to give me strength and courage. I had lost our home. My credit was in shambles. My housecleaning business worried me, could I support myself on my income, would my body hold up to the grueling pace? I was scared to look ahead to my future.

My life looked bleak and I felt alone. The loss of my sweet husband pierced my heart. I had lost myself; I had always been courageous in the face of disaster, resilient and positive. The loss of Wanda happened slowly; one-step down at a time. I hardly noticed myself disappearing in the haze of endless hours of tender caregiving. I lived only for Joe. His every wish, his every need superseded any need I may have felt. I fell asleep that night awash in tears, punctuated by deep and silent sobs.

The next morning I woke up to puffy eyes and a sluggish, heavy feeling in my legs. I stood in the shower letting the hot water run over my body and as I stood there, I could feel Joe. I began to feel his energy and a sense of wonder long since forgotten. Stay in the moment, stay in the moment was all I could hear. Feel this moment now, Wanda. Feel yourself breathe, feel my love around you like a cloak. How could I have forgotten that simple, but vital truth? Joe's legacy for me, what a gift, however for a gift to be received you must accept it. I was not alone and I had hope, if I could stay in the moment.

My mom invited me into her home and I gratefully accepted. I lived with her for a year. She kept me very busy during the day. I would work in the mornings and shop with her in the afternoons, or we would play golf. We both loved to golf and it was a great way for both of us to get outdoors.

My sister, Trudy was also a constant companion; it was very hard for her to watch me grieve. Trudy had written over fifty children's poems about fruits and vegetables. She had been trying to decide how to introduce them to the public. She took me out to lunch one day and we were surprised and delighted that a local band was playing. Their music was beautiful, they were playing rock n roll. We both love music and we found ourselves beginning to relax and sing.

Along the sidewall was a display, advertising the bandleaders business, Hear the Call Music. One of his flyers advertised cutting CD's for new artists. All of a sudden, we both looked at each other and said, "Why don't we put your poems to music!"

After their first set, the band took a break and the lead singer came over to join us. We all shook hands as we introduced ourselves to him.

"Hi, my name is Otis Coen. What are you ladies doing here today?"

Trudy said, "Hi, I'm Trudy and this is my sister Wanda. We are just having lunch and loving your music."

I asked, "You record music for people, have you ever put poems to music? Trudy has written some poems and we were wondering if you could put them to music and record them for her."

Otis intrigued us; he was outgoing and happy and asked us to wait around until the next set was over, so he could take us up to his recording studio. We happily agreed. While we listened to the lively music, Trudy and I started trying to picture her poems against a musical backdrop. We were excited and nervous about how we could make this work.

We stood opened mouthed as we stepped into a new world. Otis' studio filled with recording equipment was foreign to us. I sat down in a nearby chair as Trudy and Otis began to explore the possibility of setting her poems to his music. Ideas were flying so fast, that Trudy and Otis were verbally tripping over each other. For a short time, I forgot about Joe and became completely engrossed in this magical symphony of two artists, each with their own genres coming together as one.

Finally, I could wait no longer and I asked, "How much is this going to cost?"

Otis gave us a figure by the hour; I had the exact amount of cash in my wallet for four hours. Without thinking, I reached in my purse and pulled out the money, handed it to Otis and before Trudy could say a word, I said. "Here, this is for the first four hours!"

Trudy could not believe it, she said, "I haven't decided if I am going to do this!"

"Try four hours, and then you'll know, take a chance! I'm betting on you."

That was the day Trudy World Wide Music was born. That, was the day I began to heal. I went to every recording session with Trudy and Otis; we became a musical family. I believe fate led us to that outdoor café that magical day. The results were two CD's.

I am delighted and proud to introduce to you, Trudy's Farmer Market Kids Fall in Love with Veggies and Trudy's Farmer Market Kids Fall in Love with Fruits.

I urge you to go to Trudy's web site for more information about her, and her CD's. www.trudytunes.com. Her lyrical songs written beautifully are uplifting and appropriate for all age groups. The marriage of those two minds that fateful day was inspired; each song has a message and is unique. You and your family will find yourselves singing and dancing to the toe-tapping beats. I could not be prouder of Trudy. She set out with a dream and followed her heart to its fruition. Otis Coen will be a friend for life. Please go to his web site, *www.hearthecallmusic.com.* if he can be of service to you at your next party.

It was time for me to get back into the game of life and sadly, I knew I needed to move out of my mom's house and back into a home of my own. I jumped into action. Cheryl and I rented a house together. We spent days and weeks feathering our new little nest, without our dear husbands, but secure in the knowledge that we had each other. We jokingly referred to ourselves as the widows' Proost. Our house quickly became our home and refuge. Filled with laughter, love and sometimes tears, but always hope. We spent endless hours talking and reminiscing about our lives with Jim and Joe. We started over.

It was in that home that this book was born, with God's help and Joe looking over my shoulder. I began to write and with each passing day, I climbed up those stairs. One by one, moment by moment I began to heal.

I finally reached the top of the stairs and I found Wanda. I saw light and love, hope and the promise of life renewed and my heart raced with excitement. I realized that Joe and I walked a path that many have walked before and that many more will walk in the future. I will love again, I will cry again, I will watch loved ones struggle; I will struggle. That is the human condition. I am blessed and I bless everyone who has ever loved and lost. Those that have had to climb up those stairs alone. Rest assured that you are never truly alone, your faith and love never die.

"Remember to look up when you can't feel your feet and live life moment by moment." You can quote me!

This is Joe's legacy; this is my wish for you.

Acknowledgements

$\mathcal{M}$om, you gave me life, watched me grow, watched me love and struggle. You have always been a source of love and comfort; I love you. Thank you for urging me to start my cleaning business, thank you for loving Joe, you have always been my soft place to fall. I measure all of my accomplishments by your life well lived.

My two sisters, Trudy and Cheryl, thank you for all of your support. Trudy, thank you for your music, you gave me refuge in your beautiful songs and kept my head up when I wanted to crawl in bed and not leave. The gifts of love you both have showered on me; cannot be duplicated. I love you both very much. You walked the hard road with me and never stopped praying for us. Thank you for loving Joe.

Amy and Abby, you are the frosting of my life. You keep me on track, and you fill my life with laughter, love and a deep friendship, that is indescribable. I cannot imagine my life without both of you. When I look at you, I see me only better. You have taught me how to speak my mind and love, "Like a mad woman on wild fire!" and, "To the moon and back!" Thank you for loving and caring for Joe.

Bailey, you were there with me holding my hand as I fell in love with Joe. You were my first granddaughter and a constant source of love. I love you very much. Through your eyes, I see the world as brand new with the hope and promise of a bright future.

Joe was not only your step-grandfather, but also your great uncle. He loved you very much, thank you for showing him your love. When you wake up to "first light", he will be there for you.

Harlyn, my sweet young granddaughter, I love you so much. You came into my life when I was losing hope. On those days when life was hard, I only had to look into your innocent, young face, to be reminded of the promise of a life renewed. You held my hand as I walked Joe down those stairs. Thank you for loving JoJo, he loved you so much, he will smile down on you with pride forever.

Matt and Raechael, thank you for sharing your dad with me. The words in this book do not come close to the feelings I have for your father. I am proud and honored to have you as a part of my family. Your dad loved you beyond all measure. His love for you was unconditional and all encompassing. The miles that separated you on this earth did not separate you from his love. You each have beautiful souls and my wish for you is to live your lives in light and love. Each breath you take on this earth honors your dad and the love you shared with him.

Lloyd, we were married for twenty-five years and you know me so well. Thank you for all of your support. You were very good to Joe and I know he respected you. Thank you for the beautiful children we share and the continued love and friend-ship we enjoy. Thank you for everything.

To all the rest of my family, brothers, nieces, nephews, sons-in-laws, sister-in-laws and dear friends, I say this; I am so blessed to be a part of such a loving family and community. I do not stand-alone and for that, I am humbled beyond measure. Each one of you brings your light and love into my life every day and I thank you for all of your love and support. Thank you all for loving Joe.

I would like to thank Elyse Destout; professional photographer. Your portrait of me for the back cover was exactly what I wanted. Your beautiful studio and professional and friendly attitude made me feel comfortable and right at home. Please go to Elyse's web site www.elysedestout.com for more information about her and her beautiful photos.

Thank you to my attorney, Marc Freed. Your professional input and steady manner have been invaluable to me during this project. You showed up in my life just when I needed you.

I would like to extend a very big thank you to the Alzheimer's Foundation of America. They graciously allowed me to quote from their web site. They are working tirelessly to ease the burdens of caregivers and to find a cure for this horrific disease. As more and more people are being diagnosed with Alzheimer's, it has become more important than ever to donate time and money to help them in their quest to end this suffering. Please go to their web site for more information on how you can help. www.alzfdn.org/

Made in the USA
Charleston, SC
09 August 2015